Underground
Clinical Vignettes

Pharmacology

FIFTH EDITION

Todd A. Swanson, M.D., Ph.D.
Resident in Radiation Oncology
William Beaumont Hospital
Royal Oak, Michigan

Sandra I. Kim, M.D., Ph.D.
Resident in Internal Medicine
Beth Israel Deaconess Medical Center
Harvard Medical School
Boston, Massachusetts

Medina C. Kushen, M.D.
Resident in Neurosurgery
University of Chicago Hospitals
Chicago, Illinois

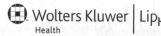 Wolters Kluwer | Lippi......
Health

Philadelphia • Baltimore • New York • London
Buenos Aires • Hong Kong • Sydney • Tokyo

Acquisitions Editor: Nancy Anastasi Duffy
Developmental Editor: Kathleen H. Scogna
Managing Editor: Nancy Hoffmann
Marketing Manager: Jennifer Kuklinski
Associate Production Manager: Kevin P. Johnson
Designer: Doug Smock
Compositor: International Typesetting and Composition
Printer: R.R. Donnelley & Son—Crawfordsville

**QV
18.2
P5364
2008**

351 West Camden Street
Baltimore, MD 21201

530 Walnut Street
Philadelphia, PA 19106

The publisher is not responsible (as a matter of product liability, negligence, or otherwise) for
any injury resulting from any material contained herein. This publication contains information
relating to general principles of medical care that should not be construed as specific instruc-
tions for individual patients. Manufacturers' product information and package inserts should
be reviewed for current information, including contraindications, dosages, and precautions.

Printed in the United States of America

First Edition, 2001 Blackwell Publishing Inc.
Second Edition, 2003 Blackwell Publishing Inc.
Third Edition, 2005 Blackwell Publishing Inc.
Fourth Edition, 2005 Blackwell Publishing Inc.

Library of Congress Cataloging-in-Publication Data

Swanson, Todd A.
    Pharmacology / Todd Swanson, Sandra Kim, Medina C. Kushen.—5th ed.
        p. ; cm.—(Underground clinical vignettes)
    Rev ed. of: Pharmacology / Vikas Bhuhan . . . [et al.]. 4th ed. c2005.
    Includes bibliographical references and index.
    ISBN-13: 978-0-7817-6485-8
    ISBN-10: 0-7817-6485-8
    1.   Clinical pharmacology—Case studies.   2.   Physicians—Licenses—United
States—Examinations—Study guides.   I. Kim, Sandra.   II. Kushen, Medina C.
III. Title.   IV. Series.
    [DNLM: 1.   Pharmacology—Case Reports.   2.   Pharmacology—Problems and
Exercises.   QV 18.2 S972p 2008]
RM301.28.P48 2008
615'.1076—dc22

                                                                            2007001467

*The publishers have made every effort to trace the copyright holders for borrowed material. If they
have inadvertently overlooked any, they will be pleased to make the necessary arrangements at the
first opportunity.*

To purchase additional copies of this book, call our customer service department at **(800) 638-
3030** or fax orders to **(301) 223-2320.** International customers should call **(301) 223-2300.**

Visit Lippincott Williams & Wilkins on the Internet: http://www.LWW.com. Lippincott Williams
& Wilkins customer service representatives are available from 8:30 am to 6:00 pm, EST.

07 08 09 10
1 2 3 4 5 6 7 8 9 10

dedication

M.K.: For my parents

preface

First published in 1999, the Underground Clinical Vignettes series has provided thousands of students with a highly effective review tool as they prepare for medical exams, particularly the USMLE Step 1 and 2 exams. Designed as a quick study guide, each UCV book contains patient-centered clinical cases that highlight a range of medical diagnoses.

With this new edition of Underground Clinical Vignettes, we have incorporated feedback from medical students across the country to provide updated cases with expanded treatment and discussion sections. A new two-page format enables readers to formulate an initial diagnosis prior to reading the answer, while the added differential diagnosis section encourages critical thinking about comparable cases. The inclusion of relevant MRI images, x-rays, and photographs allows students to more readily visualize the physical presentation of each case. Breakout boxes, tables, and algorithms have been added, along with all new Board-format QAs, making this edition of UCV an ideal source of information for exam review, classroom discussion, or clinical rotations.

The clinical vignettes in this series are designed to give added emphasis to pathogenesis, epidemiology, management, and complications. Although each case tends to present all the signs, symptoms, and diagnostic findings for a particular illness, patients generally will not present with such a "complete" picture either clinically or on a medical examination. Cases are not meant to simulate a potential real patient or an exam vignette.

Access to LWW's online companion site, ThePoint, will be offered as a premium with the purchase of the Underground Clinical Vignettes Step 1 bundle. Benefits include an online test link and additional new Board-format questions covering all UCV subject areas.

We hope you will find the Underground Clinical Vignettes series informative and useful. We welcome any feedback, suggestions, or corrections you have about this series. Please contact us at LWW.com/medstudent.

contributors

Series Editors

Todd A. Swanson, M.D., Ph.D.
Resident in Radiation Oncology
William Beaumont Hospital
Royal Oak, Michigan

Sandra I. Kim, M.D., Ph.D.
Resident in Internal Medicine
Beth Israel Deaconess Medical Center
Harvard Medical School
Boston, Massachusetts

Series Contributors

Olga E. Flomin, M.D.
Resident in Obstetrics and Gynecology
William Beaumont Hospital
Royal Oak, Michigan

Medina C. Kushen, M.D.
Resident in Neurosurgery
University of Chicago Hospitals
Chicago, Illinois

Marc J. Glucksman, Ph.D.
Professor of Biochemistry and Molecular Biology
Director, Midwest Proteome Center and
Co-Director, Rosalind Franklin Structural Biology Laboratories
Rosalind Franklin University of Medicine and Science
The Chicago Medical School
North Chicago, Illinois

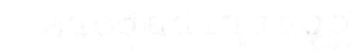

acknowledgments

Thanks to Dr. Alvaro Martinez, Dr. Larry Kestin and the entire radiation oncology program at William Beaumont Hospital for allowing the flexibility to work on this project during an already vigorous residency training program.

—Todd A. Swanson

Thanks to Todd for his work on this series.

—Sandra I. Kim

I would like to thank Todd Swanson and Sarah Lynch for helping me with this project.

—Medina C. Kushen

abbreviations

ABGs	arterial blood gases
ABPA	allergic bronchopulmonary aspergillosis
ACA	anticardiolipin antibody
ACE	angiotensin-converting enzyme
ACL	anterior cruciate ligament
ACTH	adrenocorticotropic hormone
AD	adjustment disorder
ADA	adenosine deaminase
ADD	attention deficit disorder
ADH	antidiuretic hormone
ADHD	attention deficit hyperactivity disorder
ADP	adenosine diphosphate
AFO	ankle-foot orthosis
AFP	α-fetoprotein
AIDS	acquired immunodeficiency syndrome
ALL	acute lymphocytic leukemia
ALS	amyotrophic lateral sclerosis
ALT	alanine aminotransferase
AML	acute myelogenous leukemia
ANA	antinuclear antibody
Angio	angiography
AP	anteroposterior
APKD	adult polycystic kidney disease
aPTT	activated partial thromboplastin time
ARDS	adult respiratory distress syndrome
5-ASA	5-aminosalicylic acid
ASCA	antibodies to *Saccharomyces cerevisiae*
ASO	antistreptolysin O
AST	aspartate aminotransferase
ATLL	adult T-cell leukemia/lymphoma
ATPase	adenosine triphosphatase
AV	arteriovenous, atrioventricular
AZT	azidothymidine (zidovudine)
BAL	British antilewisite (dimercaprol)
BCG	bacille Calmette-Guérin
BE	barium enema
BP	blood pressure
BPH	benign prostatic hypertrophy
BUN	blood urea nitrogen
CABG	coronary artery bypass grafting
CAD	coronary artery disease
CaEDTA	calcium edetate
CALLA	common acute lymphoblastic leukemia antigen
cAMP	cyclic adenosine monophosphate
C-ANCA	cytoplasmic antineutrophil cytoplasmic antibody
CBC	complete blood count
CBD	common bile duct
CCU	cardiac care unit
CD	cluster of differentiation
2-CdA	2-chlorodeoxyadenosine
CEA	carcinoembryonic antigen
CFTR	cystic fibrosis transmembrane conductance regulator
cGMP	cyclic guanosine monophosphate
CHF	congestive heart failure
CK	creatine kinase
CK-MB	creatine kinase, MB fraction
CLL	chronic lymphocytic leukemia
CML	chronic myelogenous leukemia
CMV	cytomegalovirus
CN	cranial nerve
CNS	central nervous system
COPD	chronic obstructive pulmonary disease
COX	cyclooxygenase
CP	cerebellopontine
CPAP	continuous positive airway pressure
CPK	creatine phosphokinase
CPPD	calcium pyrophosphate dihydrate
CPR	cardiopulmonary resuscitation
CREST	calcinosis, Raynaud phenomenon, esophageal involvement, sclerodactyly, telangiectasia (syndrome)
CRP	C-reactive protein
CSF	cerebrospinal fluid

CSOM	chronic suppurative otitis media	EMG	electromyography
CT	cardiac transplant, computed tomography	ENT	ears, nose, and throat
		EPVE	early prosthetic valve endo-carditis
CVA	cerebrovascular accident		
CXR	chest x-ray	ER	emergency room
d4T	didehydrodeoxythymidine (stavudine)	ERCP	endoscopic retrograde cholan-giopancreatography
DCS	decompression sickness	ERT	estrogen replacement therapy
DDH	developmental dysplasia of the hip	ESR	erythrocyte sedimentation rate
		ETEC	enterotoxigenic *E. coli*
ddI	dideoxyinosine (didanosine)	EtOH	ethanol
DES	diethylstilbestrol	FAP	familial adenomatous polyposis
DEXA	dual-energy x-ray absorp-tiometry	FEV_1	forced expiratory volume in 1 second
DHEAS	dehydroepiandrosterone sulfate	FH	familial hypercholesterolemia
DIC	disseminated intravascular coagulation	FNA	fine-needle aspiration
		FSH	follicle-stimulating hormone
DIF	direct immunofluorescence	FTA-ABS	fluorescent treponemal antibody absorption test
DIP	distal interphalangeal (joint)		
DKA	diabetic ketoacidosis	FVC	forced vital capacity
DL_{CO}	diffusing capacity of carbon monoxide	G6PD	glucose-6-phosphate dehydro-genase
DMSA	2,3-dimercaptosuccinic acid	GABA	gamma-aminobutyric acid
DNA	deoxyribonucleic acid	GERD	gastroesophageal reflux disease
DNase	deoxyribonuclease	GFR	glomerular filtration rate
2,3-DPG	2,3-diphosphoglycerate	GGT	gamma-glutamyltransferase
dsDNA	double-stranded DNA	GH	growth hormone
DSM	Diagnostic and Statistical Manual	GI	gastrointestinal
		GnRH	gonadotropin-releasing hor-mone
dsRNA	double-stranded RNA		
DTP	diphtheria, tetanus, pertussis (vaccine)	GU	genitourinary
		GVHD	graft-versus-host disease
DTPA	diethylenetriamine-penta-acetic acid	HAART	highly active antiretroviral therapy
DTs	delirium tremens	HAV	hepatitis A virus
DVT	deep venous thrombosis	Hb	hemoglobin
EBV	Epstein-Barr virus	HbA-1C	hemoglobin A-1C
ECG	electrocardiography	HBsAg	hepatitis B surface antigen
Echo	echocardiography	HBV	hepatitis B virus
ECM	erythema chronicum migrans	hCG	human chorionic gonadotropin
ECT	electroconvulsive therapy	HCO_3	bicarbonate
EEG	electroencephalography	Hct	hematocrit
EF	ejection fraction, elongation factor	HCV	hepatitis C virus
		HDL	high-density lipoprotein
EGD	esophagogastroduodenoscopy	HDL-C	high-density lipoprotein-cholesterol
EHEC	enterohemorrhagic *E. coli*		
EIA	enzyme immunoassay	HEENT	head, eyes, ears, nose, and throat (exam)
ELISA	enzyme-linked immunosorbent assay		
		HELLP	hemolysis, elevated LFTs, low platelets (syndrome)
EM	electron microscopy		

HFMD	hand, foot, and mouth disease	LDH	lactate dehydrogenase
HGPRT	hypoxanthine-guanine phospho-ribosyltransferase	LDL	low-density lipoprotein
		LE	lupus erythematosus (cell)
5-HIAA	5-hydroxyindoleacetic acid	LES	lower esophageal sphincter
HIDA	hepato-iminodiacetic acid (scan)	LFTs	liver function tests
HIV	human immunodeficiency virus	LH	luteinizing hormone
HLA	human leukocyte antigen	LMN	lower motor neuron
HMG-CoA	hydroxymethylglutaryl-coenzyme A	LP	lumbar puncture
		LPVE	late prosthetic valve endocardi-tis
HMP	hexose monophosphate		
HPI	history of present illness	L/S	lecithin-sphingomyelin (ratio)
HPV	human papillomavirus	LSD	lysergic acid diethylamide
HR	heart rate	LT	labile toxin
HRIG	human rabies immune globulin	LV	left ventricular
HRS	hepatorenal syndrome	LVH	left ventricular hypertrophy
HRT	hormone replacement therapy	Lytes	electrolytes
HSG	hysterosalpingography	Mammo	mammography
HSV	herpes simplex virus	MAO	monoamine oxidase (inhibitor)
HTLV	human T-cell leukemia virus	MCP	metacarpophalangeal (joint)
HUS	hemolytic-uremic syndrome	MCTD	mixed connective tissue disorder
HVA	homovanillic acid		
ICP	intracranial pressure	MCV	mean corpuscular volume
ICU	intensive care unit	MEN	multiple endocrine neoplasia
ID/CC	identification and chief complaint	MI	myocardial infarction
		MIBG	meta-iodobenzylguanidine (radioisotope)
IDDM	insulin-dependent diabetes mellitus		
		MMR	measles, mumps, rubella (vaccine)
IFA	immunofluorescent antibody		
Ig	immunoglobulin	MPGN	membranoproliferative glomeru-lonephritis
IGF	insulin-like growth factor		
IHSS	idiopathic hypertrophic subaor-tic stenosis	MPS	mucopolysaccharide
		MPTP	1-methyl-4-phenyl-tetrahy-dropyridine
IM	intramuscular		
IMA	inferior mesenteric artery	MR	magnetic resonance (imaging)
INH	isoniazid	mRNA	messenger ribonucleic acid
INR	International Normalized Ratio	MRSA	methicillin-resistant *S. aureus*
IP_3	inositol 1,4,5-triphosphate	MTP	metatarsophalangeal (joint)
IPF	idiopathic pulmonary fibrosis	NAD	nicotinamide adenine dinu-cleotide
ITP	idiopathic thrombocytopenic purpura		
		NADP	nicotinamide adenine dinu-cleotide phosphate
IUD	intrauterine device		
IV	intravenous	NADPH	reduced nicotinamide adenine dinucleotide phosphate
IVC	inferior vena cava		
IVIG	intravenous immunoglobulin	NF	neurofibromatosis
IVP	intravenous pyelography	NIDDM	non-insulin-dependent diabetes mellitus
JRA	juvenile rheumatoid arthritis		
JVP	jugular venous pressure	NNRTI	non-nucleoside reverse tran-scriptase inhibitor
KOH	potassium hydroxide		
KUB	kidney, ureter, bladder	NO	nitric oxide
LCM	lymphocytic choriomeningitis	NPO	nil per os (nothing by mouth)

NSAID	nonsteroidal anti-inflammatory drug	PO_2	partial pressure of oxygen
Nuc	nuclear medicine	PPD	purified protein derivative (of tuberculosis)
NYHA	New York Heart Association	PPH	primary postpartum hemorrhage
OB	obstetric		
OCD	obsessive-compulsive disorder	PRA	panel reactive antibody
OCPs	oral contraceptive pills	PROM	premature rupture of membranes
OR	operating room		
PA	posteroanterior	PSA	prostate-specific antigen
PABA	para-aminobenzoic acid	PSS	progressive systemic sclerosis
PAN	polyarteritis nodosa	PT	prothrombin time
P-ANCA	perinuclear antineutrophil cytoplasmic antibody	PTH	parathyroid hormone
		PTSD	post-traumatic stress disorder
PaO_2	partial pressure of oxygen in arterial blood	PTT	partial thromboplastin time
		PUVA	psoralen ultraviolet A
PAS	periodic acid Schiff	PVC	premature ventricular contraction
PAT	paroxysmal atrial tachycardia	RA	rheumatoid arthritis
PBS	peripheral blood smear	RAIU	radioactive iodine uptake
PCO_2	partial pressure of carbon dioxide	RAST	radioallergosorbent test
		RBC	red blood cell
PCOM	posterior communicating (artery)	REM	rapid eye movement
		RES	reticuloendothelial system
PCOS	polycystic ovarian syndrome	RFFIT	rapid fluorescent focus inhibition test
PCP	phencyclidine		
PCR	polymerase chain reaction	RFTs	renal function tests
PCT	porphyria cutanea tarda	RHD	rheumatic heart disease
PCTA	percutaneous coronary transluminal angioplasty	RNA	ribonucleic acid
		RNP	ribonucleoprotein
PCV	polycythemia vera	RPR	rapid plasma reagin
PDA	patent ductus arteriosus	RR	respiratory rate
PDGF	platelet-derived growth factor	RSV	respiratory syncytial virus
PE	physical exam	RUQ	right upper quadrant
PEFR	peak expiratory flow rate	RV	residual volume
PEG	polyethylene glycol	SaO_2	oxygen saturation in arterial blood
PEPCK	phosphoenolpyruvate carboxykinase		
		SBFT	small bowel follow-through
PET	positron emission tomography	SCC	squamous cell carcinoma
PFTs	pulmonary function tests	SCID	severe combined immunodeficiency
PID	pelvic inflammatory disease		
PIP	proximal interphalangeal (joint)	SERM	selective estrogen receptor modulator
PKU	phenylketonuria		
PMDD	premenstrual dysphoric disorder	SGOT	serum glutamic-oxaloacetic transaminase
PML	progressive multifocal leukoencephalopathy	SIADH	syndrome of inappropriate antidiuretic hormone
PMN	polymorphonuclear (leukocyte)	SIDS	sudden infant death syndrome
PNET	primitive neuroectodermal tumor	SLE	systemic lupus erythematosus
		SMA	superior mesenteric artery
PNH	paroxysmal nocturnal hemoglobinuria	SSPE	subacute sclerosing panencephalitis

SSRI	selective serotonin reuptake inhibitor
ST	stable toxin
STD	sexually transmitted disease
T2W	T2-weighted (MRI)
T_3	triiodothyronine
T_4	thyroxine
TAH-BSO	total abdominal hysterectomy–bilateral salpingo-oophorectomy
TB	tuberculosis
TCA	tricyclic antidepressant
TCC	transitional cell carcinoma
TDT	terminal deoxytransferase
TFTs	thyroid function tests
TGF	transforming growth factor
THC	tetrahydrocannabinol
TIA	transient ischemic attack
TLC	total lung capacity
TMP-SMX	trimethoprim-sulfamethoxazole
tPA	tissue plasminogen activator
TP-HA	*Treponema pallidum* hemagglutination assay
TPP	thiamine pyrophosphate
TRAP	tartrate-resistant acid phosphatase
tRNA	transfer ribonucleic acid
TSH	thyroid-stimulating hormone
TSS	toxic shock syndrome
TTP	thrombotic thrombocytopenic purpura
TURP	transurethral resection of the prostate

TXA	thromboxane A
UA	urinalysis
UDCA	ursodeoxycholic acid
UGI	upper GI
UPPP	uvulopalatopharyngoplasty
URI	upper respiratory infection
US	ultrasound
UTI	urinary tract infection
UV	ultraviolet
VDRL	Venereal Disease Research Laboratory
VIN	vulvar intraepithelial neoplasia
VIP	vasoactive intestinal polypeptide
VLDL	very low density lipoprotein
VMA	vanillylmandelic acid
V/Q	ventilation/perfusion (ratio)
VRE	vancomycin-resistant enterococcus
VS	vital signs
VSD	ventricular septal defect
vWF	von Willebrand factor
VZV	varicella-zoster virus
WAGR	Wilms tumor, aniridia, genitourinary abnormalities, mental retardation (syndrome)
WBC	white blood cell
WHI	Women's Health Initiative
WPW	Wolff-Parkinson-White syndrome
XR	x-ray
ZN	Ziehl-Neelsen (stain)

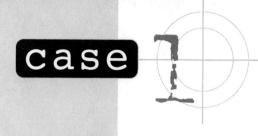

case 1

ID/CC   A 45-year-old female complains of **fatigue**, headache, dizziness, dry cough, **shortness of breath**, and **unexplained anxiety**.

HPI   She has been receiving an anti-arrhythmic medication for 1 year for treatment of chronic paroxysmal atrial fibrillation.

PE   VS: **bradycardia** (HR 55); BP normal; **diffuse crackling sounds and wheezes** in both lung fields, predominantly in bases; violaceous skin discoloration in sun-exposed areas.

Labs   ECG: **prolonged Q-T interval** and QRS duration. **AST and ALT moderately elevated.**

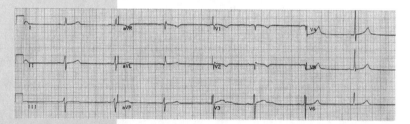

Figure 1-1. Prolonged Q-T interval in lead V3.

Imaging   CXR: bilateral interstitial infiltrates.

1

case 1

Amiodarone Side Effects

Differential

Asthma

Bronchitis

GERD

Congenital prolonged Q-T syndrome

Discussion

Amiodarone is a class III anti-arrhythmic drug. Adverse reactions require careful monitoring and include **thyroid dysfunction** (both hypo- and hyperthyroidism), **constipation, hepatocellular necrosis,** and **pulmonary fibrosis,** which may be fatal. It may also produce **bradycardia** and **heart block** in susceptible individuals. Amiodarone has a **long half-life,** so if toxicity occurs, it persists long after the drug has been discontinued. Amiodarone increases the blood levels of digoxin, phenytoin, and warfarin.

Breakout Point

> Drugs that cause pulmonary fibrosis and subsequent restrictive lung disease:
> - Bleomycin
> - Amiodarone
> - Busulfan

Treatment

Discontinue amiodarone; monitor Q-T interval until normal; steroids may be indicated for pulmonary toxicity; monitor LFTs and TFTs until they normalize after cessation of amiodarone use.

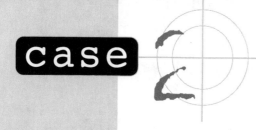

case

ID/CC A 54-year-old obese male who is the owner of a chain of fast-food restaurants is brought to the ER after **fainting at work**; earlier in the morning he complained of **dizziness and dyspnea**.

HPI He had been having episodes of acute, severe retrosternal chest pain associated with exercise or stress for over 2 years and is taking **medication for his heart**.

PE VS: **hypotension (BP 85/60); bradycardia** (HR 52). PE: lung fields have **scattered wheezes**.

Labs ECG: QRS normal, but **P-R interval increased**; [bradycardia]

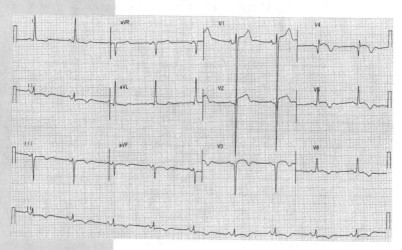

Figure 2-1. Marked bradycardia.

3

case 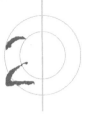2

Beta-Blocker Overdose

Differential

Dehydration
Vasovagal episode
Cardiogenic shock
Pulmonary edema

Discussion

Propranolol is a competitive nonselective beta-blocker that acts at both β_1 and β_2 receptors. β_2 receptors are found in bronchiolar and vascular smooth muscle. Uses include management of hypertension and tachyarrhythmias, hypertrophic cardiomyopathy, prevention of angina and migraines, reduction of mortality after myocardial infarction, and treatment of glaucoma and hyperthyroidism. Overdose can present with cardiac conduction disturbances, severe CNS toxicity (seizures, coma), and hyperkalemia.

Breakout Point

> Propranolol is one of the most lipid-soluble beta-blockers; as such it is used primarily for its CNS effects. It is used for **essential tremors** and **performance anxiety.**

Treatment

Treat bradycardia with atropine or epinephrine. Treat **bronchospasm** with bronchodilators. Treat hypotension with fluids and norepinephrine. Glucagon can be life-saving in this situation.

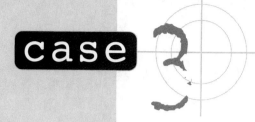

case

ID/CC   A 62-year-old woman is referred to a pulmonary medicine specialist by her family physician because of a **chronic dry cough** that has been **unresponsive to medications.**

HPI   On careful, directed questioning, the specialist discovers that she had been taking **an antihypertensive medication** for 3 years. She also complains of **taste changes** and a **rash** on her chest and lower legs.

PE   VS: normal. PE: discrete nonpruritic maculopapular **rash** on legs and chest.

Labs   Serum **renin increased; angiotensin II decreased.** Lytes: hyperkalemia. UA: mild **proteinuria.**

Imaging   CXR: no signs of COPD, neoplasm, or other pathology that would account for cough.

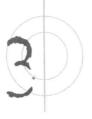

case 3

Captopril Side Effects

Differential

Asthma

Bronchitis

Hay fever

Discussion

Captopril is an ACE inhibitor and thus reduces levels of angiotensin II and prevents the inactivation of bradykinin (a potent vasodilator). It is used to treat hypertension, CHF, and diabetic renal disease. It is **contraindicated in pregnancy** because of fetotoxicity; other side effects are **cough, hypotension, taste changes, rash, proteinuria, hyperkalemia, angioedema,** and **neutropenia.**

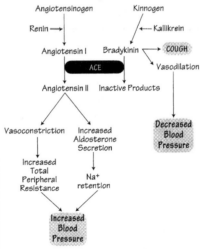

Figure 3-1. Renin-angiotensin system.

Breakout Point

> ACE inhibitors have been shown to decrease mortality in patients who have had a myocardial infarction.

Treatment

Aspirin, nifedipine, or cromolyn may decrease cough. However, it may be necessary to switch to another antihypertensive. **Losartan** is an alternative agent that blocks the binding of angiotensin II to its receptor and does not cause cough.

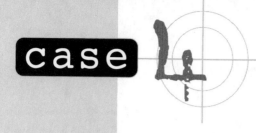

case

ID/CC   A 54-year-old white woman complains of **intermittent nausea and vomiting, headaches, lethargy,** and **confusion** over the past 3 months.

HPI   She describes objects as **appearing yellow** to her. She has a history of heart failure and takes an inotropic anti-arrhythmic medication.

PE   VS: **bradycardia** (HR 48); BP normal.

Labs   Lytes: **hypokalemia.** Elevated BUN; elevated creatinine. ECG: **AV block with AV junctional rhythm.**

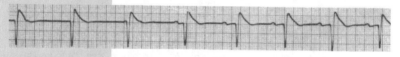

Figure 4-1. Atrioventricular (AV) junctional rhythm with first-degree AV block.

Imaging   CXR: moderate enlargement of the heart (due to long-standing CHF).

case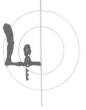

Digitalis Intoxication

Differential

Migraine headache

Brain mass

Hyponatremia

Syncope

Subdural hematoma

Discussion

Digoxin is a cardiac glycoside that inhibits the Na-K ATP-ase of cell membranes, causing an increase in intracellular sodium that results in an elevation in the intracellular calcium level, thereby causing positive inotropy. **Renal failure may precipitate toxicity** at normal therapeutic doses (excretion is decreased). Hypokalemia is a frequent predisposing factor for toxicity. ECG changes may vary widely; AV conduction disturbances, such as PAT with block, are characteristic, as are bigeminy, bradycardia, and flattened T-waves.

Breakout Point

> Digibind is a Fab fragment antibody administered in cases of digoxin toxicity. It binds and inactivates circulating digoxin

Treatment

Lower and space apart the dose. Correct hypokalemia. Digoxin-specific Fab antibody fragments.

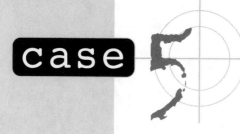

case 5

ID/CC An anesthesiologist is summoned into the OR when a 34-year-old man undergoing a **routine hernia repair** begins to have **seizures.**

HPI The surgeon was chatting with the chief resident while injecting a local anesthetic when the patient suddenly started having tremors and **tonic-clonic convulsions.**

PE Lips and fingertips blue (CYANOSIS); patient **biting his tongue;** eyes rolled inward; spastic extremities and spine with shaking movements during intervals.

Labs There was no time to take blood samples.

case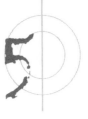

Lidocaine Toxicity

Differential

Seizure disorder

Arrhythmia

Conversion disorder

Anaphylaxis

Discussion

Lidocaine is an amide that blocks sodium channels, primarily in rapidly firing cells such as those in the myocardium, in pain fibers, and in the CNS. Overdosage occurs with inadvertent systemic injection, mainly in obstetric and surgical procedures, and is manifested by CNS toxicity (seizures) and a "hyper" state. This is **followed by a depressive period** with obtundation, hypotension, and **cardiorespiratory depression**. Toxicity should be differentiated from the infrequent anaphylactic reaction.

Treatment

Control seizures with IV diazepam or barbiturates. Intubate, oxygenate, and ventilate in anticipation of second phase (respiratory depression).

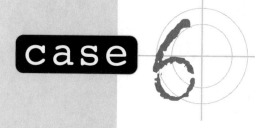

ID/CC A 52-year-old man visits his physician complaining of **extreme tiredness, dry mouth, and easy fatigability**; he states that he has never experienced symptoms such as these before.

HPI He was started on hydrochlorothiazide for treatment of hypertension, but it did not control his hypertension, so a new medication was added approximately 2 months ago. On directed questioning, he states that he has been suffering from **sexual dysfunction** for the past several weeks.

PE VS: BP 130/90, but when standing up it is 100/60; bradycardia (HR 58). PE: **conjunctival pallor.**

Labs CBC: **positive Coombs test;** decreased hemoglobin and hematocrit; **increased reticulocytes and spherocytes; decreased haptoglobin.** UA: hemoglobinuria. Increased indirect bilirubin; normal iron levels.

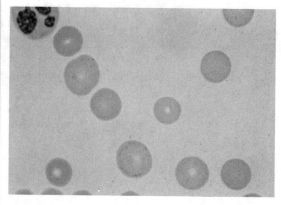

Figure 6-1. Spherocytes from patient with autoimmune hemolytic anemia.

Imaging CXR/KUB: normal for age.

case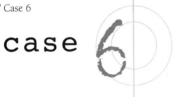

Methyldopa Side Effects

Differential

Cancer

Dehydration

Diabetes

B-blocker side effects

Hemolytic anemia

Discussion

Methyldopa is a sympatholytic that produces a false neurotransmitter, α-methyl-norepinephrine, which activates inhibitory $\alpha2$-receptors in the CNS. It is used as an antihypertensive drug, and its side effects include **impotence, Coombs positivity** (20% of patients), and, more rarely, **hemolytic anemia.** It can also cause **sedation, drowsiness,** severe orthostatic hypotension, and hepatic toxicity.

Breakout Point

The Coombs test is used to detect the presence of antibodies bound to red blood cells (RBCs). Complement is added to RBCs during the test. Lysis by complement indicates that the cells had auto-antibodies bound to them.

Treatment

Switch antihypertensive treatment.

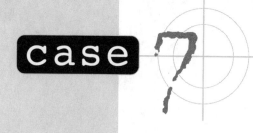

case 7

ID/CC The 48-year-old chief executive officer of a leading auto manufacturer is put on **a new medication** and a restricted diet for the treatment of **high-LDL cholesterol.**

HPI On a visit 2 months afterward, the patient's lab tests show improvement, but he complains of **facial flushing** and **itching** on the lower back, palms, and anus.

PE VS: mild hypertension (BP 145/95). PE: obesity; **face, neck, and chest flushed**; no skin rash demonstrable on inspection.

Labs **Serum glucose elevated (157 mg/dL); LDL lowered** considerably in comparison to last visit; **triglycerides decreased,** but not as markedly; **HDL increased; AST and ALT** mildly **elevated; elevated uric acid;** normal levels of 5-hydroxyindoleacetic acid.

Imaging CXR: normal.

case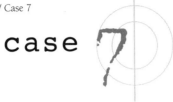

Niacin Side Effects

Differential | Carcinoid syndrome
Liver disease
Serotonin syndrome
Erythema nodosum

Discussion | Nicotinic acid (NIACIN) is a derivative of tryptophan, a constituent of NAD and NADP that is used in redox reactions. As a drug, it is used for its lipid-lowering properties (decreases VLDL, decreases LDL, and increases HDL cholesterol). **Hepatitis, hyperglycemia,** and exacerbation of peptic ulcer are other side effects.

■ TABLE 7-1 AGENTS USED TO TREAT LIPID DISORDERS

Drug Class	Drugs	Mechanism of Action	Major Side Effects
HMG CoA reductase inhibitors	*Atorvastatin* *Fluvastatin* *Lovastatin* *Pravastatin* *Simvastatin*	Inhibits HMG CoA reductase	Rhabdomyolysis, myoglobinuria, renal dysfunction
Fibric acid derivates (fibrates)	*Gemfibrozil* *Clofibrate* *Fenofibrate*	Inhibit lipolysis and the hepatic secretion of VLDL	Myositis when taken with statins
Nicotinic acid	*Niacin*	Inhibits VLDL synthesis and secretion	Skin flushing and pruritus
Bile acid resins	*Cholestyramine* *Colestipol*	Binds bile acids in the gut	Constipation, heartburn, nausea

Breakout Point

> **Drugs that cause cutaneous flushing on administration:**
> - Niacin
> - Calcium channel blockers
> - Adenosine
> - Vancomycin

Treatment | Flushing and itching are often transient. Aspirin diminishes symptoms by inhibiting prostaglandin synthesis.

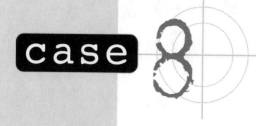

case 8

ID/CC	A 53-year-old man who works in a **chemical factory** presents with **chronic headaches and dizziness** with occasional **chest pain.**
HPI	The patient states that his headaches and dizziness occur most frequently when he **returns to work** after a few days off; he is otherwise in good health.
PE	PE: patient appears normal but **slightly cyanotic;** lung fields clear.
Labs	**Methemoglobin levels elevated.** ECG: no sign of ischemia or necrosis.
Imaging	CXR/KUB: within normal limits for age.

case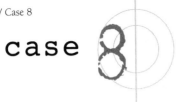

Nitrate Exposure

Differential | Hyperventilation syndrome
Pulmonary embolism
Carbon monoxide poisoning
Acute anemia

Discussion | Nitrates are a large class of drugs that are used in treatment of angina. All agents in this group, including nitroglycerin, act through nitric oxide (NO) release. NO, in turn, is a potent vasodilator of vascular smooth muscle. These compounds have a short half-life and may **produce tolerance in chronically exposed individuals.** Patients may suffer **angina or MI** as a result of **rebound coronary vasoconstriction** due to withdrawal.

Breakout Point

> Nitric oxide (NO) is also known as endothelial-derived relaxation factor (EDRF)

Treatment | Avoid exposure. Methylene blue to act as electron donor for NADPH-methemoglobin reductase.

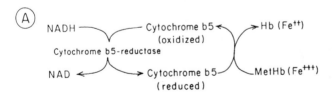

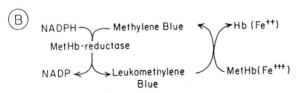

Figure 8-1. Pathways in methemoglobin (MetHb) reduction.

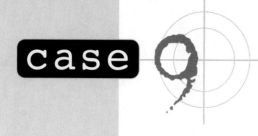

ID/CC A 56-year-old male comes to the cardiology unit for evaluation of **ringing in his ears, dizziness, GI distress** (nausea, vomiting, and diarrhea), and **headaches.**

HPI He also complains of **blurred vision** and **impaired hearing.** The patient had an MI 1 year ago and has been receiving oral anti-arrhythmic therapy.

PE VS: **bradycardia** (HR 55); BP normal (BP 110/70). PE: funduscopic exam normal but **accommodation impaired; skin flushed;** hands show fine **tremors.**

Labs CBC: normal. Lytes: normal. ECG: **prolonged Q-T interval.**

Imaging CXR: no pulmonary edema.

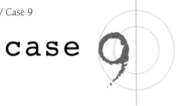

case 9

Quinidine Side Effects

Differential
Ménière disease

Benign paroxysmal vertigo

Discussion
Quinidine, procainamide, and disopyramide are class IA anti-arrhythmics that act by **blocking sodium channels, increasing the effective refractory period.** They are used for both atrial and ventricular arrhythmias. All these agents have low therapeutic-toxic ratios and may produce severe adverse reactions. **Cinchonism** is commonly produced by drugs that are cinchona derivatives, such as quinidine and quinine. The effects may occur with only one dose.

Breakout Point

> Drugs that prolong the Q-T interval can ultimately cause torsade de pointes arrythmias. In addition to class IA anti-arrhythmics, other common offending agents include:
> - Erythromycin
> - Haloperidol
> - Cisapride

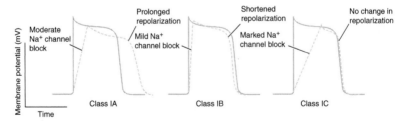

Figure 9-1. Effects of class IA anti-arrhythmics on ventricular action potential.

Treatment
Monitor ECG and vital signs; change to different anti-arrhythmic drug. Treat cardiotoxic effects with sodium lactate.

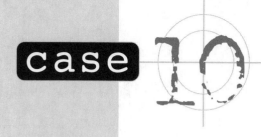

ID/CC A 73-year-old widow visits her cardiologist complaining of **difficulty moving her bowels** for the past week; she also reports **facial flushing.**

HPI She had been regular until she began taking **an antiarrythmic medication** for an irregular heartbeat 1 month ago.

PE VS: heart rate normal; BP normal. PE: abdomen soft and nondistended; mild lower leg **edema.**

Labs CBC/Lytes/UA: normal. BUN, normal levels of 5-hydroxyindoleacetic acid.

Imaging CXR: within normal limits for age. KUB: moderate amount of stool; no sign of obstruction.

case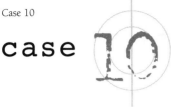

Verapamil Side Effects

Differential

Carcinoid syndrome

Hypercalcemia

Hypothyroidism

Discussion

Verapamil is one of the agents that block voltage-dependent calcium channels, consequently reducing muscle contractility. Verapamil acts more specifically on myocardial fibers than on arteriolar smooth muscle. It is widely used as an antihypertensive, as an anti-arrhythmic agent, and for treatment of angina pectoris. **Constipation** is a common side effect; other side effects include dizziness, facial **flushing,** hyperprolactinemia, and peripheral edema.

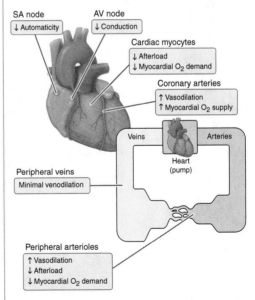

Figure 10-1. Sites of action of calcium channel blockers.

Treatment

Increase fluids in diet, regular exercise, fruits, high-bulk foods, or bulk laxatives. If persistent, change to another calcium channel blocker.

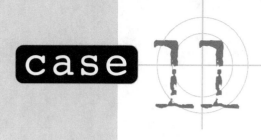
ID/CC   A 19-year-old woman is admitted to the internal medicine ward because of **generalized desquamation** of the skin, high **fever**, and painful **ulcers and bullae in her eyes and vagina.**

HPI   She adds that **swallowing** is extremely **painful.** For the past week, she has been on oral **antibiotics** for a urinary tract infection.

PE   VS: **fever** (39.2°C). PE: painful **mucosal ulcerations** in conjunctiva, nose, mouth, oropharynx, and vagina; eyelids swollen and erythematous; **generalized, symmetric rash** on skin with **macules, papules, vesicles,** and **bullae** as well as areas of denudation (epidermis completely separated from dermis) on palms, soles, and extremities.

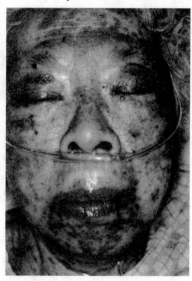

Figure 11-1. Patient on presentation.

Micropathology   Dermal edema with perivascular inflammatory infiltrate and epidermal separation in bullae showing necrotic and hemorrhagic areas.

DERMATOLOGY

21

case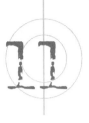

Stevens–Johnson Syndrome

Differential

Pemphigus

Toxic epidermal necrolysis

Chemical burn

Scalded skin syndrome

Discussion

Also called **erythema multiforme major**, Stevens–Johnson syndrome is a grave, acute, and sometimes fatal disease with generalized skin **desquamation** and severe **ulcers and bullae** on at least two mucosal surfaces, including the genitalia, mouth, conjunctiva, nose, or lips. The use of sulfa drugs (bacteriostatic antibiotics, which are PABA antimetabolites that inhibit dihydropteroate synthase) is a common precipitating factor. Other drugs implicated are **phenytoin,** penicillins, and barbiturates.

Breakout Point

> Drugs that commonly are associated with the development of Stevens–Johnson syndrome:
> - Phenytoin
> - Sulfonamides
> - Ethosuximide
> - Lamotrigine

Treatment

Hospitalization, discontinue sulfa drug, prophylactic antibiotics (due to increased risk of infections acquired through large areas of denuded skin), barrier nursing, antihistamines. Steroids have not been demonstrated to be effective.

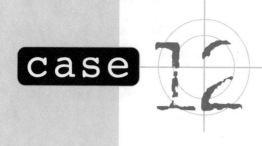

case 12

ID/CC   A 32-year-old man who works as a professional weight lifter comes to the family medicine clinic for evaluation of **impotence** for the past 4 months.

HPI   His girlfriend reports increasingly **aggressive** and **labile behavior.**

PE   VS: **borderline hypertension.** PE: young, muscular male; androgenic **alopecia; acne; gynecomastia; testicular atrophy.**

Labs   CBC/Lytes: normal. **Hyperglycemia** (145 mg/dL); **oligospermia** on semen analysis.

Imaging   Normal.

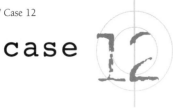

case **12**

Anabolic Steroid Abuse

Differential
Mood disorder
Erectile dysfunction.
Testicular neoplasm

Discussion
Anabolic steroids are widely abused by weight lifters, other athletes, and the lay public. Although androgens increase muscle mass significantly, they produce only slight increases in strength. Numerous side effects have been reported, including **hepatic neoplasia, glucose intolerance, decreased HDL-C levels, hypertension, testicular atrophy and oligospermia, virilization and amenorrhea, acne,** and **alopecia.** Other consequences of androgen abuse include mood disturbances and **irritability** that may result in **aggressive behavior** and injury to others.

■ **TABLE 12-1 ADVERSE EFFECTS OF ANDROGEN REPLACEMENT THERAPY**

	Virilizing Effects	Feminizing Effects[a]	Toxic Effects[b]
Women	• Acne • Facial hair • Deepening of voice • Menstrual irregularities • Male-pattern baldness • Altered musculature • Hypertrophy of the clitoris • Masculinization of female embryos following in utero exposure		• Edema • Jaundice and cholestatic hepatitis[c] • Peliosis hepatitis • Hepatic carcinoma • Skewing of diagnostic tests
Children	• Premature closure of the epiphyseal plates • Altered bone development		
Men	• Inhibition of gonadotropin release • Reduce spermatogenesis lasting months after discontinuation	Gynecomastia	

[a]Exacerbated in children and men with poor liver function.
[b]All patients.
[c]Especially with the 17-α alkyl substituted androgens.

Treatment
Discontinue androgens.

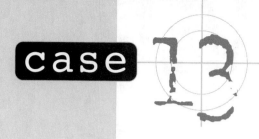

ID/CC A 46-year-old woman comes to the medical clinic for an evaluation of **weight gain, roundness of her face,** and epigastric pain that is relieved by eating.

HPI She had been suffering from chronic, itchy blisters in the mouth that came and went, leaving painful ulcers together with large bullae on all four extremities and on her chest and lower back (PEMPHIGUS), for which she has been taking **an immune suppressive medication** for several months.

PE VS: hypertension (BP 145/95). PE: **moon facies, acne, buffalo hump, truncal obesity, striae, increased facial hair,** and **ecchymoses** on distal extremities.

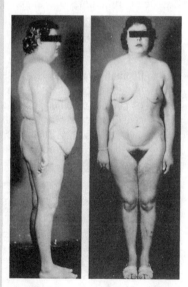

Figure 13-1. Patient at presentation.

Labs CBC: leukocytosis with **lymphopenia. Hyperglycemia.** Lytes: **hypokalemia.** UA: glycosuria.

Imaging XR, spine and long bones: generalized **osteoporosis.**

case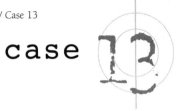

Cushing Syndrome—Iatrogenic

Differential

Obesity

Hypothyroidism

Alcoholism

Diabetes

Discussion

Of the causes of Cushing syndrome, iatrogenesis is the most common. Steroids produce a lysosomal membrane stabilization, blocking leukotriene formation from arachidonic acid, blocking the action of phospholipase A, and inhibiting cyclooxygenase activity (decreased prostaglandin formation). Because of this, steroids are used in a number of settings, such as acute inflammation, anaphylaxis, allergy states, and immune suppression as well as for the treatment of Addison disease.

Breakout Point

> **Cushing syndrome** is a disease caused by an excess of cortisol production or by excessive use of cortisol or other similar steroid (glucocorticoid) hormones. **Cushing disease** is the name given to a type of Cushing syndrome caused by too much ACTH production in the pituitary.

Treatment

Institute steroid-sparing agents such as methotrexate, azathioprine, dapsone, or nicotinamide. Corticosteroids should be tapered down.

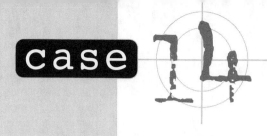
ID/CC A 32-year-old woman comes for her first gynecologic visit.

HPI On routine pelvic exam a vaginal **mass** is felt. The **patient's mother took an estrogen compound** during pregnancy as treatment for threatened abortion.

PE Well developed with breast tissue appropriate to age; pubic and axillary hair normal; on bimanual pelvic examination a **hard, ulcerated mass** is felt on posterior **wall of upper vagina**; iodine staining of vaginal wall shows patches of decreased uptake by cells (due to adenosis).

Labs CBC/Lytes/UA: normal. Hormonal screen and LFTs do not disclose any abnormality.

Imaging Hysterosalpingogram: injection of contrast into uterine cavity reveals T-shaped uterus and cervical incompetence.

Micropathology Biopsy by colposcopy shows glandular epithelium in upper part of vagina with squamous metaplasia (ADENOSIS). Biopsy of the ulcerated mass shows **clear-cell adenocarcinoma of vagina**.

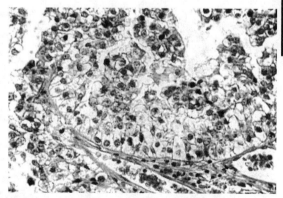

Figure 14-1. Clear cells.

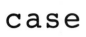
case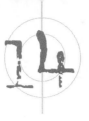

Diethylstilbestrol (DES) Exposure

Differential

Squamous cell carcinoma of the vagina

Cervical cancer

Uterine cancer

Uterine fibroids

Discussion

Diethylstilbestrol is a synthetic estrogen that was used some 30 to 35 years ago for the prevention of a threatened abortion. The daughters of patients thus treated before the 18th week of pregnancy may present with an alteration in the development of the embryonic transition between the urogenital canal and paramesonephric system, producing persistence of the müllerian glands on the upper vagina and giving rise to adenosis and clear cell adenocarcinoma that is usually asymptomatic and discovered incidentally. Other side effects include transverse vaginal septum, developmental uterine abnormalities, and cervical incompetence. In males DES may be associated with genital tract abnormalities.

Treatment

Surgery; radiation.

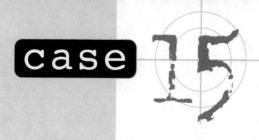
ID/CC A 36-year-old female oboe player is brought by ambulance to the emergency room because of gradual numbness and **weakness on the left side of her face and arm** along with **headache** and dizziness.

HPI She is **obese** and **smokes** one pack of cigarettes a day. She is currently sexually active and uses appropriate measures to prevent pregnancy.

PE VS: normal. PE: patient conscious, oriented, and able to speak; **gaze is deviated to the right;** funduscopic exam does not show papilledema, hypertension, or diabetic retinopathy; left **arm and leg weakness with hyporeflexia.**

Labs CBC/Lytes: normal. ECG: normal.

Imaging CT, head: negative. Arteriography: thrombotic cerebral arterial occlusion.

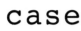 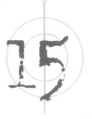

Oral Contraceptive Side Effects

Differential

Seizure

Brain mass

Encephalitis

Discussion

Oral contraceptive pills are a very popular method of birth control. There are many OCP preparations; most consist of a combination of estrogens and progestins which, when taken daily, selectively inhibit pituitary function to prevent ovulation. The most severe complication is an **increased incidence of vascular thrombotic events,** either cerebral or myocardial. Other side effects include nausea, acne, weight gain, psychological depression, cholestatic jaundice, increased incidence of vaginal infections, headaches, and breakthrough bleeding. OCPs should be used cautiously in patients with asthma, diabetes, liver disease, and hypertension.

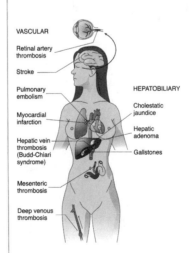

Figure 15-1. Complications of oral contraceptives.

Treatment

Intensive care treatment and surveillance for stroke in evolution. Evaluate anticoagulation, discontinue OCPs.

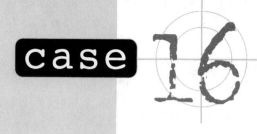

case 16

ID/CC	A **55-year-old, postmenopausal** white **woman** complains of **nausea, headaches, weight gain, and breast tenderness.**
HPI	She was placed on **hormonal medication** 6 months ago and is also taking **calcium** and **vitamin D**. She had a **hysterectomy** 5 years ago. There is no history of breast, uterine, or ovarian cancer in her family.
PE	VS: normal. PE: mild tenderness to palpation over lumbar vertebrae; breast exam reveals diffuse tenderness without any palpable masses; no axillary lymphadenopathy.
Labs	Lipid profile reveals decreased LDL, increased HDL, and elevated triglycerides.
Imaging	X-ray of spine: thinning of the spine and prominence of the cortex. DEXA: **osteopenia** in thoracolumbar vertebral bodies.

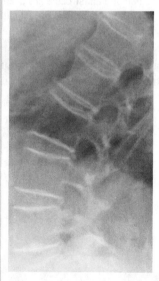

Figure 16-1. Generalized bone demineralization.

ENDOCRINOLOGY

31

case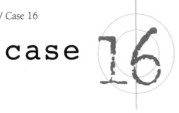

Osteoporosis Prophylaxis—Hormonal

Differential

Perimenopausal symptoms

Discussion

Until recently, estrogen replacement therapy (ERT) was considered to be first-line therapy for post-menopausal osteoporosis prophylaxis. In patients with an intact uterus, hormone replacement therapy (HRT) included progesterone to reduce the risk of endometrial cancer. Results from the Women's Health Initiative (WHI) trial confirmed risk reduction of osteoporotic fractures in women on ERT or HRT but found an increased risk for stroke and pulmonary embolism (ERT) as well as coronary artery disease and breast cancer (HRT). Current guidelines are evolving but tend to encourage nonhormonal treatment for the prevention of chronic disease, including osteoporosis.

Breakout Point

> Estrogen-blocking compounds such as tamoxifen and anastrozole are used in the treatment of hormone-sensitive breast cancers.

Treatment

Discontinue estrogens and strongly consider use of nonhormonal agents (e.g., bisphosphonates, calcitonin) for long-term osteoporosis prophylaxis.

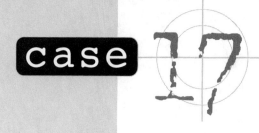

case 17

ID/CC A **53-year-old, postmenopausal woman** presents to the outpatient clinic with questions regarding "that bone disease" and requests a bone density scan.

HPI She drinks at least three cups of **coffee and smokes** a pack of cigarettes daily. She is married with two children. There is no history of alcohol abuse, corticosteroid use, or osteoporosis among immediate family members. She **strongly refuses any oral prophylactic hormone therapy.**

PE VS: normal. PE: unremarkable.

Imaging DEXA: mild **osteopenia.**

case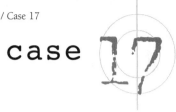

Osteoporosis Prophylaxis—Nonhormonal

Discussion

Osteoporosis is a bone disease characterized by a decrease in bone density. It is classically a disease of **elderly, thin, postmenopausal Caucasian** or **Asian females** and commonly causes hip and vertebral fractures. Hip fractures can occur secondary to a **fall** but also result from repetitive stress on the hip during intensive exercise programs. **Smoking** increases the risk of osteoporosis, but **caffeine** intake is now believed to have minor or no effect on bone density or fractures. Low to moderate intake of **alcohol** is beneficial, as it increases estrogen levels. **Multiparity** is protective. Calcium is believed to **decrease bone resorption,** probably by inhibiting PTH secretion, but is far less potent than **estrogen** in preventing osteoporosis. Metabolites of **vitamin D** increase the intestinal absorption of calcium, and the most active metabolite, **calcitriol,** or $(1,25)$ OH_2 vitamin D, stimulates bone formation via osteoblasts.

Breakout Point

> Despite all the ill effects of obesity, the one thing that it seems to be protective for is the development of osteoporosis. This is presumably due to the increased production of estrogens in adipose tissue.

Treatment

Calcium and **vitamin D supplementation;** regular **exercise and a balanced diet;** counsel on **fall prevention** and **smoking cessation;** alternative therapy with **bisphosphonates,** selective estrogen receptor modulators (**SERMs**), and **calcitonin.**

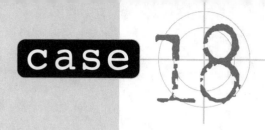

case 18

ID/CC 67-year-old, **postmenopausal white woman** presents with **weakness, muscular twitching,** and a nagging **retrosternal heartburn.**

HPI She was placed on **preventative osteoporosis therapy** 6 months ago following the diagnosis of a **spinal compression fracture** secondary to advanced osteoporosis. She is **not on any calcium or vitamin D supplementation.**

PE VS: normal. PE: carpopedal spasm noted on inflating BP cuff (TROUSSEAU'S SIGN); facial twitching noted on tapping anterior to the tragus (CHOVSTEK'S SIGN); spinal kyphosis and protuberant abdomen.

Labs Lytes: **hypocalcemia. Elevated PTH levels.**

ENDOCRINOLOGY

case 18

Osteoporotic Fracture—Bisphosphonates

Differential

Angina pectoris

GERD

Gastritis

Discussion

Bisphosphonates such as **alendronate** and **pamidronate** increase bone mass by decreasing bone resorption. Side effects include **hypocalcemia, increased PTH levels,** and **upper GI irritation/ esophageal ulceration** when given orally. Other medications given for osteoporosis include **raloxifene, a selective estrogen receptor modulator (SERM),** and **calcitonin.** Calcitonin causes increases in bone density (not as much as seen with bisphosphonates) and is a safe alternative to estrogen. Side effects include nasal irritation when administered as a nasal spray.

Breakout Point

> Several of the intravenous preparations of the various bisphosphonates are approved for the treatment of bony metastasis in cases of breast or prostate cancer.

Treatment

Calcium replacement with vitamin D; advise patient to **take alendronate in upright posture** to reduce reflux and risk of esophagitis; H_2 blockers or proton pump inhibitors for concomitant or exacerbated peptic ulcer disease/GERD.

case 19

ID/CC A **37-year-old obese man** presents with recent worsening of his anginal symptoms.

HPI He suffers from **coronary artery disease** and regularly takes anti-anginal medications. One month ago, he began to take a **stimulant-containing supplement** for weight loss and to "increase his energy level."

PE VS: borderline **hypertension** (BP 150/100).

Labs ECG: normal.

Imaging CXR: normal.

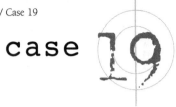

case

Alternative Pharmacotherapy

Differential
Unstable angina
Myocardial infarction
GERD

Discussion
Herbal supplements as alternative medicines are currently in widespread use. Over 20% of the general population use herbal supplements for health, but fewer than 50% of those taking supplements tell their physician. **Ephedrine (Ma Huang)** is a sympathomimetic drug that stimulates the sympathetic nervous system and is synergistic with **caffeine.** The adverse effects of ephedrine include **increased blood pressure, palpitations, chest pain, psychosis, tremor, insomnia, dry mouth,** and **cardiomyopathy** linked to chronic use.

Treatment
Stop ephedrine-containing supplement and educate on risks of unsupervised use of herbal/alternative medicines; evaluate for worsening coronary artery disease if symptoms do not abate after stopping the supplement.

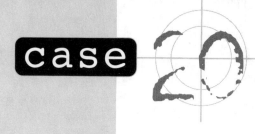

case 20

ID/CC	A **36-year-old white morbidly obese woman** presents to her primary care physician, seeking help with losing weight.
HPI	She has tried various diets and exercise programs with no success.
PE	VS: normal. PE: morbidly obese.
Labs	CBC/Lytes: normal. Lipid panel, LFTs, TSH normal.

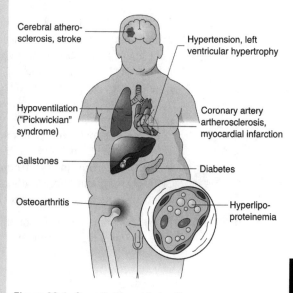

Figure 20-1. Complications of obesity.

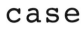

case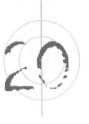

Anorectic/Anti-Obesity Agents

Discussion

Obesity contributes to **atherosclerosis, CAD, hyper-lipidemia, hypertension, and type II diabetes.** Anti-obesity drugs currently on the market include **orlistat** and **sibutramine.** They are indicated for weight loss and maintenance in conjunction with a calorie-reduced diet in patients with a body mass index >30. Orlistat is a **lipase inhibitor** that acts in the GI tract and **blocks the absorption of dietary fat.** The most common adverse effects are GI-related and include spotting, flatus, and fatty stools. Absorption of lipid-soluble vitamins (e.g., vitamin K) or medications (e.g., griseofulvin) may be decreased. Sibutramine treats obesity through **appetite suppression;** it acts centrally by blocking serotonin and nor-epinephrine reuptake. Adverse effects include headache, dry mouth, constipation, insomnia, and a **substantial increase in blood pressure and heart rate in some patients.** Sibutramine is contraindicated in patients on MAO inhibitors or SSRIs (may precipitate **serotonin syndrome**), in those with CHF/CAD, and in those with hepatic dysfunction (the drug is metabolized by **cytochrome P450).**

Treatment

Orlistat or **sibutramine** in combination with a structured diet and exercise program.

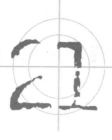

case 21

ID/CC	A 64-year-old man with **metastatic lung cancer** is seen with complaints of **severe bone pain, anorexia,** and **cachexia.**
HPI	He spends most of his time in bed because of profound weakness and chronic nausea.
PE	VS: **mild fever** (38.0°C); **tachycardia** (HR 110); **underweight** (45 kg, body mass index 17). PE: **cachetic; sunken eyes; prominent skin wrinkles/folds; visible loss of significant skeletal muscle mass.**

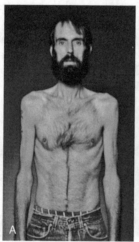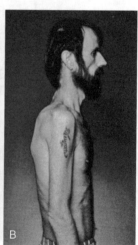

Figure 21-1. Cachexia.

Labs	CBC: lymphopenia. Lytes: **hypokalemia; hypochloremia.** ABGs: **metabolic alkalosis.** Decreased albumin and prealbumin/transthyretin.

case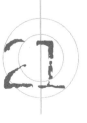

Appetite Stimulants—Megestrol/THC

Differential

AIDS

Anorexia

Malabsorption syndrome

Discussion

Cachexia/anorexia syndrome is characterized by progressive weight loss, lipolysis, loss of muscle mass, anorexia, diarrhea, and fever in patients with end-stage cancer or AIDS. Some drugs that have proven effective in improving appetite and treating cachexia include **megestrol acetate** and **dronabinol.** Megestrol is a synthetic progesterone that stimulates the appetite, resulting in weight gain and recovery of muscle mass. It is relatively nontoxic. Side effects are rare and include **altered menses with unpredictable bleeding** and **mild edema.** Dronabinol, a synthetic **tetrahydrocannabinol (THC),** is the active component in **marijuana** and is used to treat nausea and vomiting associated with cancer chemotherapy as well as to stimulate appetite. Side effects are due mainly to the psychoactive effects of the drug and include dizziness, ataxia, hallucinations/psychosis, tachycardia, hypertension, and URI symptoms.

Breakout Point

> Weight loss in patients with cancer is predominately caused by the systemic production of tumor necrosis factor (TNF)-α, also known as cachexin.

Treatment

Treat with **megestrol acetate or dronabinol** to increase appetite; adequate palliative pain medications.

ID/CC A 35-year-old man presents to his family doctor because of increasing embarrassment and concern over **breast enlargement**.

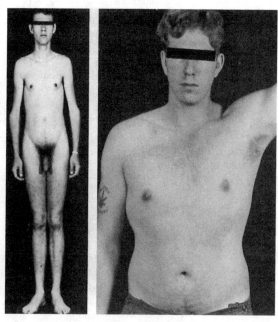

Figure 22-1. Moderate gynecomastia.

HPI The patient has a long history of burning epigastric pain on awakening in the mornings and between meals that decreases with food and antacids (peptic ulcer disease), for which he has been taking **cimetidine**. Directed questioning reveals that he has also been suffering from **impotence**.

PE VS: normal. PE: moderate bilateral growth of breast tissue; **testes** somewhat **hypotrophic**.

Labs CBC/Lytes/UA: normal.

Imaging CXR/KUB: normal.

GASTROENTEROLOGY

43

case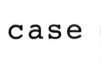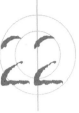

Cimetidine Side Effects

Differential
Pituitary neoplasm
Weight gain
Anabolic steroid side effects
Cushing syndrome

Discussion
All the H_2-blockers are well tolerated, although cimetidine is associated with several side effects, particularly **reversible gynecomastia.** H_2-blockers produce an **increase in serum prolactin levels** (especially ranitidine) and alter estrogen metabolism in men (have anti-androgenic properties). Other side effects include headache, confusion, low sperm counts, and hematologic abnormalities (thrombocytopenia may enhance hypoprothrombinemic effect of oral anticoagulants). They have been largely supplanted by newer H_2-receptor blockers without many of these side effects.

Breakout Point

> Commonly used drugs that cause gynecomastia, as they compete for androgen receptors:
> • Cimetidine
> • Ketoconazole
> • Sprirolactone

Treatment
Switch to other histamine receptor antagonists, such as ranitidine or famotidine.

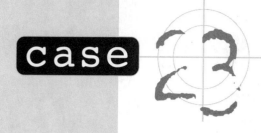

case 23

ID/CC	A 58-year-old woman comes to the emergency room because of acute, burning **epigastric pain** accompanied by nausea and **vomiting** of **bright red blood**.
HPI	She is a chronic sufferer of rheumatoid arthritis and has taken an anti-inflammatory pain medication every 8 hours for the past 4 years to control her pain.
PE	VS: **tachycardia** (HR 98); hypotension (BP 110/60). PE: **pallor;** abdomen shows **tenderness on deep palpation in epigastrium;** no rigidity, guarding, or rebound tenderness.
Labs	CBC: low hemoglobin and hematocrit.
Imaging	Endoscopy: gastric mucosa markedly hyperemic with hemorrhagic spotting and zones of recent hemorrhage; no ulcer or tumor observed.

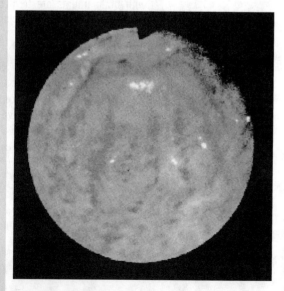

Figure 23-1. Endoscopy finding of marked hyperemia with hemorrhagic spotting.

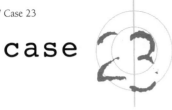

case

Hemorrhagic Gastritis—Drug-Induced

Differential

GERD

Peptic ulcer disease

Gastric cancer

Esophageal varices

Discussion

Hemorrhagic gastritis is seen in individuals who take drugs that may cause damage to gastric mucosa, such as aspirin, NSAIDs, steroids, and alcohol. Critically ill patients, such as those with burns, sepsis, cranial trauma, and coagulation defects, may also bleed from the stomach. Acetylsalicylic acid (aspirin) acetylates and irreversibly inhibits cyclooxygenase 1 and 2 to prevent conversion of arachidonic acid to prostaglandins.

Breakout Point

> The stress ulcers seen in critically ill patients with brain trauma are termed **Cushing ulcers** and those with ulcers associated with burns are known as **Curling ulcers.**

Treatment

Discontinue offending agent; give prostaglandins such as **misoprostol** that inhibit acid secretion and enhance mucosal defense; replace nonselective NSAID agents with **selective cyclooxygenase inhibitors** that spare the gastric receptors, such as celecoxib; start mucosal protectors, antacids, **proton pump inhibitors,** or H_2-receptor blockers.

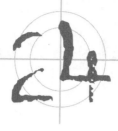

ID/CC   A 64-year-old woman is brought to the emergency room because of the development of high fever, **marked jaundice**, weakness, profound fatigue, and **darkening of her urine**.

HPI   She has undergone many surgical procedures **under general anesthesia** over the past 2 years, including endometrial biopsy, femoral hernia repair, and, 4 weeks ago, total hip replacement. After each surgery, the patient developed a low-grade fever within a few days.

PE   VS: **tachycardia** (HR 93); hypotension (BP 100/55); fever (39.2°C). PE: **marked weakness**; diaphoresis; patient appears **toxic**; profound **jaundice**; liver edge palpable 3 cm below costal margin and tender.

Labs   CBC: marked **leukocytosis** (18,500) with **eosinophilia** (18%). Hypoglycemia; **AST and ALT markedly elevated; elevated alkaline phosphatase and bilirubin.**

Gross Pathology   Massive centrolobular hepatic necrosis with fatty change.

case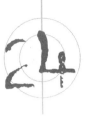

Hepatitis—Halothane

Differential

Ascending cholangitis
Biliary obstruction
Viral hepatitis
Alcoholic fatty liver
Septic shock

Discussion

All inhaled anesthetics cause a decrease in hepatic blood flow, but rarely does this result in permanent derangement of liver function tests. Nonetheless, hydrocarbon drugs that include halothane are considered hepatotoxic. Most commonly, such drugs produce elevated LFTs, but they may also cause postoperative jaundice and hepatitis. Rarely does fulminant hepatic failure result, but such failure carries a 50% mortality rate. Occurrence is normally 4 to 6 weeks after halothane exposure. Middle-aged, obese women with several halothane exposures within closely spaced intervals are most at risk.

Breakout Point

> Drugs that can cause massive hepatic necrosis:
> • Halothane
> • Acetaminophen
> • Valproic acid

Treatment

Monitor liver function; assess bilirubin, glucose levels, and PT. Provide intensive supportive care for possible hepatic failure and encephalopathy. Treat hypoglycemia with glucose, treat bleeding with fresh frozen plasma, and use lactulose to prevent encephalopathy.

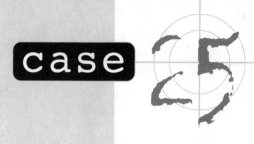

case 25

ID/CC A 52-year-old HIV-positive man who was diagnosed with **tuberculosis** and started on **antimycobacterial** therapy 8 months ago presents with **jaundice.**

HPI The patient's therapy was uneventful until 2 weeks ago, when he began to appear jaundiced. He also complains of **lack of strength and sensation in his feet.**

PE VS: normal. PE: patient appears lethargic; yellowed sclera and discoloration of skin; moderate, nontender hepatomegaly; decreased strength and diminished perception of light touch in feet.

Labs Moderately **increased AST, ALT,** and **bilirubin.**

Imaging US: generalized mild enlargement of liver with no focal lesions.

case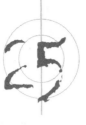

Hepatitis—INH

Differential

Viral hepatitis

Alcoholic hepatitis

Hemochromatosis

Discussion

Isoniazid (isonicotinic acid hydrazide) decreases the synthesis of mycolic acids and is the bactericidal drug of choice for tuberculosis prophylaxis. It is used as combination therapy for eradication of *Mycobacterium tuberculosis*. Chronic use is associated with **hepatitis**, **peripheral neuritis**, disulfiram-like reaction, and **systemic lupus erythematosus**. INH competes with pyridoxine for the enzyme apotryptophanase, thus producing a deficiency of pyridoxine. The administration of pyridoxine can prevent some central and peripheral nervous system effects.

Breakout Point

> Drugs that can cause a SLE-like syndrome:
> • Hydralazine
> • Procainamide
> • Isoniazid
> • Phenytoin

Treatment

More than a two- to threefold increase in AST and ALT warrants cessation of INH use. Also stop rifampin if it is part of multidrug therapy for tuberculosis. Substitution with second-line antitubercular agents (e.g., fluoroquinolones, aminoglycosides) may be required. Mild derangement of liver function warrants close monitoring while treatment with INH is continued. Co-administration of pyridoxine with INH is recommended to prevent and possibly ameliorate peripheral neurotoxicity.

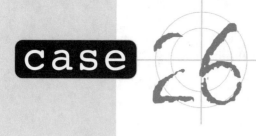

case 26

ID/CC	A 22-year-old woman presents to the ER with severe abdominal colic and a history of **profuse watery diarrhea** of several days' duration.
HPI	She also complains of **dizziness** and a **desire to lose weight** (directed questioning discloses that she has been taking a **laxative** intermittently).
PE	VS: **hypotension** (BP 80/45); no fever. PE: **skin shriveled; bowel sounds hyperactive;** oliguric and lethargic.
Labs	Lytes: hypokalemia; hyponatremia; hyperchloremia. ABGs: normal anion gap metabolic acidosis.
Micropathology	Deposition of dark pigmentation in the colonic mucosa after long-standing use of anthraquinone-containing laxatives. Termed **melanosis coli,** a misnomer as it is lipofuscin, not melanin, which accumulates in cells.

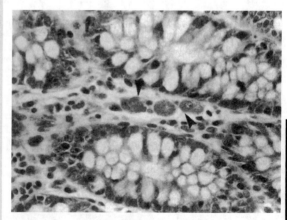

Figure 26-1. Lipofuscin-like pigment within macrophages (*arrows*) in the lamina propria of a rectal biopsy specimen from a patient with melanosis coli.

GASTROENTEROLOGY

case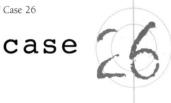

Laxative Abuse

Differential
Bacterial gastroenteritis
Viral gastroenteritis
Colitis
Malabsorption syndromes

Discussion
Laxative abuse remains a common way people attempt to lose weight; abuse is also common among psychiatric patients. Laxatives can interfere with the absorption of several medications, such as tetracycline and calcium supplements. Laxatives may act by irritating the mucosa, through direct neuronal stimulation, via an osmotic increase in the water content of stool, through softening of stool by a detergent-like action, or by forming bulk. Continued abuse may lead to melanosis coli, colonic neuronal degeneration, and the "lazy syndrome." Patients with chronic constipation abuse laxatives to the point of being dependent on them for evacuation.

Treatment
Discontinue laxatives and offer counseling; electrolyte and fluid replacement.

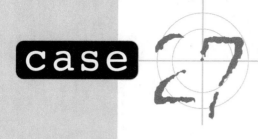

case 27

ID/CC	A 28-year-old woman has surgery due to perforated appendicitis with peritonitis; 10 days postoperatively she develops fever, abdominal cramping, and **diarrhea with pus and mucus.**
HPI	Her postoperative recovery was unremarkable until the onset of diarrhea. She had **received continuous parenteral antibiotics.**
PE	VS: fever; tachycardia; tachypnea. PE: moderate dehydration; mild abdominal tenderness with no signs of peritoneal irritation; surgical wound normal.
Labs	CBC: leukocytosis. Stool culture reveals gram-positive rods.
Imaging	Sigmoidoscopy: mucosal hyperemia, ulcers, and **pseudomembranes.**
Gross Pathology	Mucosa hyperemic and swollen; epithelial ulcerations covered by yellowish plaques (pseudomembranes) and fibrinous exudate.
Micropathology	Fibrinous exudate with pseudomembrane formation; ulceration of superficial epithelium; neutrophilic infiltrate with necrotic debris.

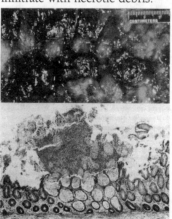

Figure 27-1. Mushroom-shaped cloud of adherent of inflammatory exudate on the colon.

GASTROENTEROLOGY

case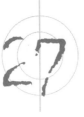

Pseudomembranous Colitis

Differential | Campylobacter infection
Amebiasis
Inflammatory bowel disease
Shigellosis
Ischemic colitis

Discussion | Pseudomembranous colitis is defined as acute inflammation of the colon in patients taking antibiotics, specifically **clindamycin** or ampicillin, due to **overgrowth of *C. difficile*;** it is characterized by formation of **pseudomembranes.** Clindamycin acts by blocking protein synthesis at the 50S ribosomal unit. Its main clinical indication is for life-threatening infections with **anaerobes.**

Breakout Point 1

> Drugs that cause significant ototoxicity and nephrotoxicity:
> - Aminoglycosides
> - Loop diuretics
> - Cisplatin

Breakout Point 2

> Commonly used antibiotics that inhibit the 30S bacterial ribosome:
> - Aminoglycosides
> - Tetracyclines
>
> Commonly used antibiotics that inhibit the 50S bacterial ribosome:
> - Chrolamphenicol
> - Erythromycin (and other macrolides)
> - Clindamycin
> - Linezolid
> - Streptogramins

Treatment | Cessation of offending antibiotic; give **metronidazole** or oral vancomycin.

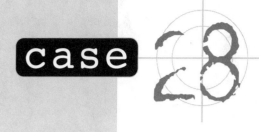

case 28

ID/CC   A 6-year-old boy is brought by his parents to the emergency room in a **comatose state**.

HPI   The child had been suffering from **chickenpox** and had been given **an anti-pyretic** by the family physician for fever.

PE   VS: **fever**. PE: comatose child with **papulovesicular rash** all over body; fundus shows **marked papilledema**; no icterus; moderate hepatomegaly; asterixis.

Labs   **Marked hypoglycemia; increased blood ammonia concentration; elevated AST and ALT; prolonged PT;** serum bilirubin normal. LP (done after lowering raised intracranial pressure): normal CSF.

Imaging   CT: findings suggestive of **generalized cerebral edema**.

Gross Pathology   Severe cerebral edema; acute hepatic necrosis.

Micropathology   Liver biopsy reveals microvesicular steatosis with little or no inflammation; electron microscopy shows marked mitochondrial abnormalities.

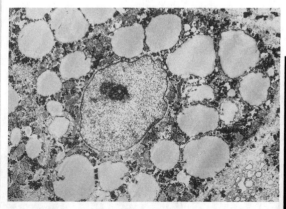

Figure 28-1. Microvesicular steatosis of hepatocytes.

GASTROENTEROLOGY

case 28

Reye Syndrome

Differential
: Encephalitis
Meningitis
Mushroom poisoning
Inborn errors in metabolism
Jamaican vomiting sickness

Discussion
: Although the cause of the highly lethal Reye syndrome (hepatoencephalopathy) is unknown, epidemiologic evidence strongly links this disorder with outbreaks of viral disease, especially influenza B and chickenpox. Epidemiologic evidence has also prompted the Surgeon General and the American Academy of Pediatrics Committee on Infectious Diseases to recommend that **salicylates not be given to children with chickenpox or influenza B.**

Treatment
: Specific therapy is not available. Supportive measures include lactulose to control hyperammonemia, fresh frozen plasma to replenish clotting factors, mannitol or dexamethasone to lower increased intracranial pressure, and mechanical ventilation. Exchange transfusion; dialysis.

case 29

ID/CC A 51-year-old chemical engineer who manages the production line at a large **petrochemical plant** comes to his family doctor for a yearly checkup; he is asymptomatic but is found to have **microscopic painless hematuria**.

HPI He is a **heavy smoker** and has been working at the production plant over a period of 25 years.

PE VS: normal. PE: strongly built male with gray hair and smoke discoloration of his mustache and finger-tips; a few wheezes heard on lung fields.

Labs CBC/Lytes: normal. Clinical chemistry and LFTs normal; BUN and creatinine normal. UA: **hematuria**.

Imaging US: no renoureteral lithiasis; no pelvicalyceal dilatation. Excretory urography: filling defect and rigidity in wall of urinary bladder.

Micropathology Urine cytology shows marked dysplastic and anaplastic transitional cells; cystoscopy and biopsy confirm a **papillary transitional cell carcinoma (TCC) of the bladder**.

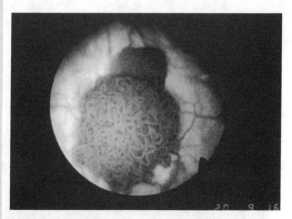

Figure 29-1. Papillary transitional-cell carcinoma of the bladder seen by cystoscopy.

57

case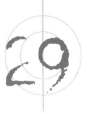

Aniline Dye Carcinogenicity

Differential

Nephrolithiasis

Nephritis

Urethritis

Renal cell carcinoma

Urinary tract infection

Discussion

The substances 2-amino-1-naphthol and p-diphenyl-amine are the two carcinogens that are presumed to be involved in the genesis of transitional cell bladder cancer in individuals exposed to **anilines**, benzidine, and **β-naphthylamines**. Saccharin has been shown to induce TCC in rats. Cigarette smoking greatly increases the risk. Heavy caffeine consumption remains a controversial risk factor.

Breakout Point

Well-known exposure and cancer associations:

Substance	Cancer
Aniline dyes	Bladder cancer
Asbestos	Mesotheliomas
Radon	Lung cancer
Arsenic	Skin cancer
Chromium and nickel	Lung cancer
Vinyl chloride	Angiosarcoma of the liver
Diethylstibesterol (DES)	Vaginal cancer
Nitrosamines (food preservatives)	Stomach cancer

Treatment

Surgery, chemotherapy, radiotherapy.

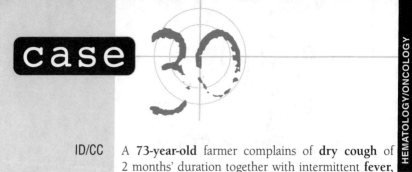

ID/CC   A **73-year-old** farmer complains of **dry cough** of 2 months' duration together with intermittent **fever, vomiting,** and increasing **dyspnea.**

HPI   He had a squamous cell carcinoma lesion surgically removed from his nose several months ago and received **chemotherapy.**

PE   Healed skin flap on left nasal fossa; no local lymphadenopathy; multiple freckles and solar dermatitis on scalp; scattered lung **rales and wheezing; soles of feet** show painful, erythematous areas with **skin thickening.**

Labs   CBC/Lytes: normal. PFTs: decreased FEV_1 and FVC with normal FEV_1/FVC ratio.

Imaging   CXR: bilateral pulmonary infiltrates but no evidence of metastatic disease.

Micropathology   Lung biopsy shows interstitial pneumonitis with fibrosis and bronchiolar squamous metaplasia.

case

Bleomycin Toxicity

Differential

Bronchiolitis obliterans organizing pneumonia
(BOOP)

Asbestosis

Radiation pneumonitis

Emphysema

Metastatic lung cancer

Discussion

Bleomycin is an antibiotic produced by *Streptomyces verticillus* that acts by DNA fragmentation. It is used in a variety of epidermoid and testicular cancers. Fever and chills may ensue with the administration of the drug by any of the parenteral routes available (it is not active orally). It has very little marrow toxicity and almost no immune suppression, but the keratinized areas of the body may suffer from hypertrophy and nail pigmentation. **Pulmonary fibrosis** is a side effect that characteristically arises in older patients and in those with preexisting lung disease.

Breakout Point

> Bleomycin is used to treat several types of cancer, including cervix and uterus cancer, head and neck cancer, testicle and penile cancer, and certain types of lymphoma. It is an important part of the **ABVD** regiment for Hodgkin lymphoma that includes **A**driamycin, **B**leomycin, **V**inblastine, and **D**acarbazine.

Treatment

Steroids, antibiotics, discontinue bleomycin.

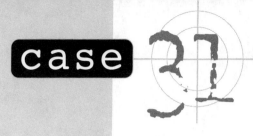

case 27

ID/CC A 20-year-old man with **testicular cancer** presents to his oncologist with a pronounced **decrease in bilateral auditory acuity.**

HPI His last two chemotherapy sessions were administered by an intern who only recently arrived at the municipal hospital.

PE VS: normal. PE: auditory testing shows bilateral **neurosensory deficit in the high-frequency range;** lung fields do not show crackles or wheezing; heart sounds rhythmic with no murmurs; neurologic exam reveals loss of **proprioception** in feet and **diminished sensation in hands and feet** (STOCKING-GLOVE PATTERN).

Labs CBC: normal. Lytes: **hypomagnesemia; hypocalcemia;** hypernatremia; hypokalemia. **BUN and creatinine increased.**

Imaging CT, head: no intracranial causes of hearing loss revealed.

case 31

Cisplatin Side Effects

Differential | Ménière disease
Ear infection
Aminoglycoside toxicity
Vancomycin toxicity
Salicylate toxicity

Discussion | Cisplatin is an effective chemotherapeutic drug that acts like an alkylating agent, cross-linking DNA via the hydrolysis of chloride groups and reaction with platinum. It is used for bladder and testicular cancers as well as for some ovarian tumors. It can produce severe **renal damage** if administered in the absence of abundant **hydration**. It also causes **CN VIII damage** with permanent deafness. Another side effect is **peripheral neuropathy.**

Treatment | Vigorous hydration and diuresis to reduce severity of aeate nephrotoxicity; electrolyte replacement; pretreatment with amifostine may reduce nephrotoxicity and neurotoxicity.

■ TABLE 31-1 CHEMOTHERAPEUTIC SIDE EFFECTS

Myelosuppressive	*Cyclophosphamide, busulfan, cisplatin, carboplatin, paclitaxel, methotrexate, cytarabine, etoposide, 6-mercaptopurine*
Non-myelosuppressive	*Vincristine, bleomycin*
Hemorrhagic cystitis	*Cyclophosphamide, ifosfamide*
Nephrotoxic	*Cisplatin, mitomycin C*
Pulmonary toxic	*Bleomycin, busulfan*
Cardiotoxic	*Doxorubicin, daunorubicin*
Neurotoxic	*Cisplatin, vincristine, paclitaxel*
Bladder cancer	*Cyclophosphamide*
Teratogenic	*Leflunomide, tamoxifen*
Allergy	*Paclitaxel*
Mouth ulcers	*Methotrexate*

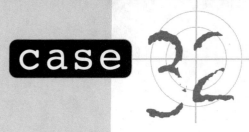

case

ID/CC   A 40-year-old man who has been diagnosed with pemphigus vulgaris complains of **dysuria** and **increased urinary frequency.**

HPI   The patient has no history of fever or gross hematuria. He is receiving monthly **chemotherapy** pulses.

PE   VS: normal. PE: no pallor; lungs clear to auscultation; cardiac exam normal; abdomen soft and nontender; no suprapubic masses; no peritoneal signs; no tenderness in costovertebral angle.

Labs   CBC: normocytic, normochromic **anemia;** mild leukopenia and thrombocytopenia. UA: **microscopic hematuria** but no bacteriuria.

case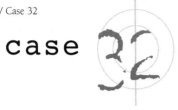

Cyclophosphamide Side Effects

Differential	UTI
	Prostatitis
	Radiation cystitis
	Renal cell carcinoma
	Interstitial cystitis

Discussion Cyclophosphamide is an alkylating agent that covalently cross-links DNA at guanine N-7 and requires bioactivation by the liver. It is used for lymphomas and for breast and ovarian carcinomas, as well as certain autoimmune conditions. Complications of cyclophosphamide use include **hemorrhagic cystitis, bladder fibrosis,** and **bladder carcinoma; sterility; alopecia;** and inappropriate ADH secretion. Cyclophosphamide needs to be converted to an active toxic metabolite, **acrolein,** which is responsible for producing hemorrhagic cystitis.

Treatment Maintain good hydration and HCO_3 loading; β-amino caproic acid and mesna may prevent hemorrhagic cystitis.

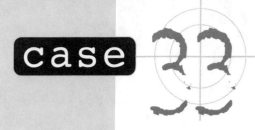

case

ID/CC	A 59-year-old woman currently being treated for **breast cancer** is brought by ambulance to the ER after fainting while at work.
HPI	The patient had noticed a painless lump in her right breast 6 months earlier. She was diagnosed with invasive ductal carcinoma on biopsy and placed on an adjuvant **chemotherapy** regimen.
PE	VS: **tachycardia** (HR 110); BP normal (118/85). PE: **elevated JVP;** S3 auscultated; **basal rales** in lung fields; **hepatomegaly; pitting edema** in lower legs.
Labs	ECG: ST-T changes, premature ventricular contractions; decreased QRS voltage.
Imaging	CXR: cardiomegaly and pulmonary congestion. Echo: dilated cardiomyopathy with reduced ejection fraction.
Gross Pathology	Increase in weight and size of heart with softened, weak walls and dilated chambers (DILATED CARDIOMYOPATHY).

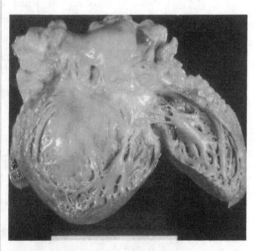

Figure 33-1. Dilated cardiomyopathy.

65

case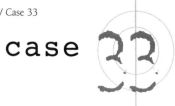

Doxorubicin Cardiotoxicity

Differential

Amyloidosis

Wet beriberi

Glycogen storage diseases

Myocarditis

Iron toxicity

Congestive heart failure

Discussion

Doxorubicin, also called adriamycin, is an anthracy-cline antibiotic that binds to DNA and blocks the synthesis of new RNA and/or DNA, thereby blocking cell replication. It is used in the treatment of carcino-mas of the ovary, breast, testicle, lung, and thyroid. It is also used in the treatment of many types of sarco-mas and hematologic cancers. Side effects are mainly cardiac but may also include alopecia and marrow toxicity (cardiomyopathy associated with doxoru-bicin is dose-related and irreversible; the mechanisms may be related to the intracellular production of free radicals in myocardium, which can be prevented by **dexrazoxane**).

Breakout Point

"The Rubin sisters, they will break your heart." Both anthracyclines, dauno**rubicin** and doxo**rubicin,** cause dose-limiting cardiotoxicity.

Treatment

Treatment of heart failure due to **dilated cardiomy-opathy.** Discontinue doxorubicin.

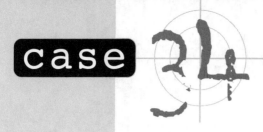

ID/CC   A **74-year-old woman** who recently had hip replacement surgery has been on **postoperative anti-clotting medication** for 5 days for the prevention of possible pulmonary embolism; shortly thereafter, she starts to have black, tarry stools (MELENA, GI BLEEDING), hematuria, and **bleeding from the gums** when brushing her teeth.

HPI   She suffers from long-standing cardiac disease and has a **history of deep venous thrombosis**.

PE   VS: no fever; **heart rate slightly elevated above baseline**; BP within normal limits but drops when patient stands up (ORTHOSTATIC HYPOTENSION). PE: **pallor**; no signs of cardiac failure; **incision is oozing blood**; venipuncture sites show large **ecchymoses**.

Labs   CBC: normocytic, normochromic **anemia** (7.3 mg/dL). **aPTT and PT markedly elevated**.

Imaging   CXR: within normal limits for age. XR, hip: no evidence of hematoma formation.

case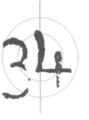

Heparin Overdose

Differential

Peptic ulcer disease

Esophagitis

Hemophilia

Disseminated intravascular coagulation

Discussion

Heparin complexes with **antithrombin III** to form a potent **inactivator of factor Xa** and **inhibitor of the conversion of prothrombin** to thrombin. This complex also inactivates factors IXa, XIa, and XIIa. Its major adverse effect is bleeding, which occurs with a higher incidence in women over age 60. Other adverse effects include hypersensitivity, hyperlipidemia, hyperkalemia, osteoporosis, and, in up to 30% of patients, thrombocytopenia. The severity of thrombocytopenia appears to be dose related and is due to the direct effect of heparin on platelets or to an immunoglobulin that aggregates platelets.

Treatment

Stop heparin; for significant bleeding complications, IV **protamine sulfate** is the specific antidote.

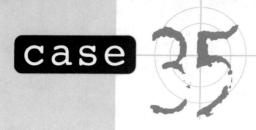

ID/CC A 9-year-old boy is brought to the emergency room after intentionally ingesting half a bottle of **supplements used for anemia** (coated with plum-flavored sugar) 6 hours ago; he now complains of **abdominal pain and diarrhea**.

HPI He has been feeling weak and lightheaded, with palpitations and a metallic taste in his mouth. He had two episodes of **bluish-green vomit** followed by a large **hematemesis**.

PE VS: marked **tachycardia** (HR 120); **hypotension** (BP 90/50); no fever. PE: pulse weak; patient is **pale and dehydrated** with cold and clammy skin; lungs clear; abdomen tender to deep palpation, predominantly in epigastrium, with no peritoneal signs; neurologic exam normal; rectal exam discloses **black, tarry stool.**

Labs Markedly elevated serum iron levels (>500 mg/dL). UA: rose-wine colored urine. ABGs: metabolic acidosis. BUN and creatinine elevated.

Imaging XR, abdomen: multiple **radiopaque tablets** in GI tract from stomach to jejunum. Endoscopy: **diffuse hemorrhagic gastritis** with extensive necrosis and sloughing of mucosa.

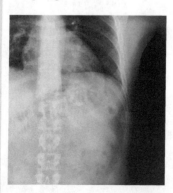

Figure 35-1. Iron-containing tablets in the left upper quadrant.

case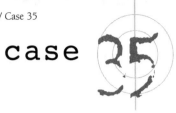

Iron Overdose

Differential

Gastroenteritis

Acetaminophen toxicity

Arsenic toxicity

Constipation

Mercury toxicity

Hemochromatosis

Discussion

Mortality due to acute iron overdose may reach 25% or more, mainly in children. There may be marked dehydration and shock.

Treatment

Gastric lavage with bicarbonate solution (to form ferrous carbonate, which is not absorbed well) or induction of vomiting. Treat acidosis; treat shock with IV fluids and **chelation** therapy with **deferoxamine.**

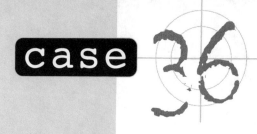

case

ID/CC   A 62-year-old woman comes to the general oncology unit of the university hospital for **ulceration of the oral mucosa and diarrhea.**

HPI   She is being treated for carcinoma of the breast with aggressive **chemotherapy.**

PE   VS: hypotension (BP 100/50); tachycardia (HR 105). PE: lethargic and dehydrated; oral mucosa and tongue show erythema and shallow ulcers (BUCCAL STOMATITIS); skin rash on volar aspect of forearms.

Labs   CBC: **anemia; thrombocytopenia; leukopenia** (myelosuppression). BUN and creatinine elevated.

case 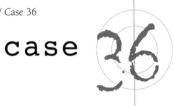 36

Methotrexate Toxicity

Differential
Behçet disease

Fungal infection

Herpes zoster

Discussion
Methotrexate binds **reversibly** with dihydrofolate reductase, preventing the synthesis of purine and pyrimidine nucleotides. The toxic effects on proliferating tissues are particularly deleterious to the bone marrow, skin, and GI mucosa. **Leucovorin** "rescue" attenuates some of these toxic effects because it is a metabolically active form of folic acid. For that reason, it does not require reduction by dihydrofolate reductase. Therefore, leucovorin has the capacity to catalyze the one-carbon transfer reactions necessary for purine and pyrimidine biosynthesis.

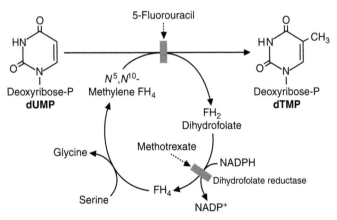

Figure 36-1. Mechanism of methotrexate.

Treatment
The efficacy of leucovorin therapy depends on early administration when methotrexate toxicity is suspected. Give IV dose equal to or greater than the dose of methotrexate.

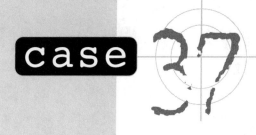

case

ID/CC A 53-year-old woman presents with **dizziness and spontaneous severe bruising.**

HPI She reports passage of several dark, tarry stools (MELENA). She underwent a valve replacement several months ago and is currently taking **an anticoagulant.** One week ago, she was given **co-trimoxazole** (a sulfa antibiotic) for a "sinus infection," but she neglected to tell her doctor about her other medications.

PE VS: **orthostatic hypotension** (BP 110/70, HR 95 when supine; BP 90/60, HR 110 when erect). PE: extensive ecchymoses and petechiae noted on skin exam; black, tarry guaiac positive stools on rectal exam.

Labs CBC: **anemia. PT, INR, PTT markedly elevated.**

case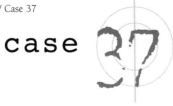

Warfarin Interactions

Differential

Peptic ulcer disease

Gastritis

Hemophilia

Discussion

Warfarin is an **anticoagulant** commonly used in patients with **underlying hypercoagulable states, prosthetic cardiac valves, cardiac arrhythmias, DVTs, and pulmonary embolism.** It acts by interfering with the hepatic synthesis of vitamin K-dependent clotting factors, resulting in depletion of factors VII, IX, X, and II. Warfarin is highly **protein bound,** primarily to albumin, and is metabolized by the hepatic **cytochrome P450 enzyme system. Drug interactions** with warfarin are extensive. They include increased effect due to inhibition of metabolism (e.g., amiodarone, cimetidine, co-trimoxazole), possible increased effect due to displacement from albumin (e.g., chloral hydrate, furosemide), and decreased effect due to induction of metabolism (e.g., barbiturates, rifampin).

Breakout Point

> Although there are a number of drugs that induce the hepatic P450 system, the more commonly encountered offenders include:
> - Phenytoin
> - Carbamazepine
> - Griseofulvin
> - Rifampin
> - Barbiturates
> - Chronic alcohol intake

Treatment

Supportive (blood transfusion and IV fluids); for significant bleeding complications associated with warfarin use (as in this case), withhold warfarin, administer **fresh frozen plasma** and parenteral **vitamin K,** and monitor serial PT/PTT/INR.

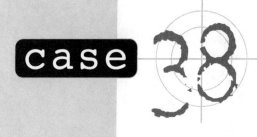

case 28

ID/CC   A 32-year-old man with a prosthetic heart valve complains to his family doctor of **black, tarry stools**.

HPI   He had been receiving **oral anticoagulation medicine** to prevent thrombus formation. Two years ago, he had an **aortic valve replacement** due to destruction of the valve secondary to bacterial endocarditis. The patient has a **hereditary deficiency of protein C**.

PE   VS: BP normal; pulse rate normal. PE: subconjunctival hemorrhage; bleeding gums; **bruises and petechiae** on arms and legs (generalized bleeding). **Necrosis of the skin.**

Labs   Stool guaiac positive. UA: hematuria. **Markedly elevated PT** (affects extrinsic coagulation pathway).

case 38

Warfarin Toxicity

Differential | Peptic ulcer disease
Gastritis
Hemophilia

Discussion | This patient has generalized bleeding, including GI tract bleeding secondary to warfarin treatment. Warfarin compounds inhibit **epoxide reductase** and hepatic production of the vitamin K-dependent clotting factors (II, VII, IX, and X), interfering with their **γ-carboxylation.** Only de novo synthesis is affected; therefore, therapy must continue for 2 to 3 days before effects are noted. Effects of warfarin last between 5 and 7 days. Warfarin crosses the placenta and is thus contraindicated in pregnant women.

Breakout Point

> Pregnant patients who need to be anticoagulated, such as those with a hypercoaguable syndrome, need to be switched to heparin, which is safe during pregnancy and does not cross the placenta.

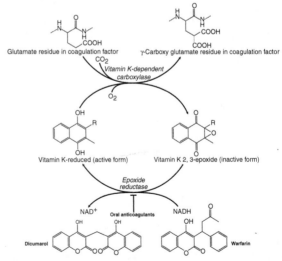

Figure 38-1. Mechanism of oral anticoagulants.

Treatment | If significant bleeding and volume depletion have occurred, consider fresh frozen plasma and transfusions. Vitamin K may be required.

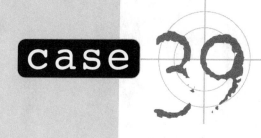

case 29

ID/CC	A 45-year-old man who received a **renal transplant** 4 months ago comes to the oncology unit for a follow-up exam complaining of headache and ringing in his ears. He was found to have **hypertension.**
HPI	He is currently taking multiple **immunosuppressive** drugs.
PE	VS: **hypertension** (BP 150/110). PE: no jaundice; no pallor; cardiac exam normal; abdomen soft and non-tender; no abdominal masses; no peritoneal signs; fine hand **tremors** at rest.
Labs	**Elevated BUN and serum creatinine.** Lytes: **hyperkalemia.** UA: **proteinuria.** ECG: peaked T-waves (hyperkalemia).
Micropathology	Renal biopsy reveals presence of tubular lesions (vacuolization), atrophy, edema, microcalcifications, and absence of an acute cellular infiltrate that is characteristic of acute rejection.

IMMUNOLOGY

case 39

Cyclosporine Side Effects

Differential

Transplant failure

Renal artery stenosis

Discussion

Cyclosporine is an immunosuppressive agent used for the prevention of rejection in organ transplantation. Subacute nephrotoxicity is the most important side effect and is frequently seen in the first weeks or months following transplantation. Other side effects include hypertension, hyperkalemia, hyperuricemia (gout), hyperglycemia, neurotoxicity (tremor, irritability, seizure), and an increased incidence of EBV-related B-cell lymphomas. Cyclosporine is metabolized in the liver by the cytochrome P450 system.

Breakout Point

> Cyclosporin inhibits the protein calcineurin, a gene needed for production of the T-cell proliferative factor, interleukin (IL)-2.

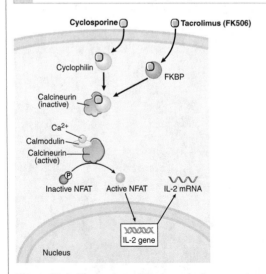

Figure 39-1. Mechanism of the immunosupressants cyclosporin and tacrolimus.

Treatment

Reduction in cyclosporine dose with serial monitoring.

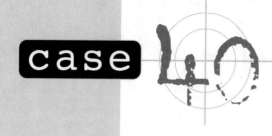

ID/CC A 58-year-old woman presents with **persistent fever, chills, headache, weakness,** and **diffuse muscle and bone aches.**

HPI She was diagnosed with **chronic myelocytic leukemia** (CML) a few months ago and is now being treated with oral hydroxyurea and subcutaneous **cytokine agent.**

PE VS: **fever** (39.0°C); **tachycardia** (HR 105). PE: appears fatigued; splenomegaly on abdominal exam.

Labs CBC: **anemia;** mild **leukopenia;** mild **thrombocytopenia.** No blast cells seen.

case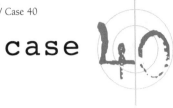

Interferon Use

Differential

Influenza infection

Pneumonia

HIV infection

Discussion

Interferons are **cytokines** with antiviral, antiprolifer-
ative, and immunomodulating properties. They are
used to treat chronic hepatitis B, C, or D infection
(α2b), condyloma acuminatum (genital warts) due to
HPV (α2b, αn3), CML or hairy-cell leukemia (α2a,
α2b), Kaposi sarcoma (α2a, α2b), melanoma (α2b),
and chronic granulomatous disease (γ2b). Side
effects include **fever, chills, myalgias, fatigue, pan-
cytopenia,** and **neurotoxicity** that presents as **somnolence** and **confusion.** Autoimmune phenomena,
including **thyroiditis** (both hypo- and hyperthyroidism), **autoimmune hemolytic anemia,** and
thrombocytopenia, can also occur secondary to
interferon use.

Treatment

In the presence of intolerable side effects, replace
interferon with alternative therapy.

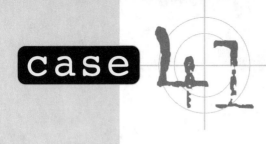

case 47

ID/CC   During ward rounds, a 28-year-old **HIV-positive** woman complains that after a period of improvement since her admission 3 days ago, she now feels very sick, with **high fever, marked lightheadedness, headache,** and **myalgias.**

HPI   She was admitted because of **cryptococcal meningitis** and was started on **antifungal medication.**

PE   VS: tachycardia (HR 93); **hypotension** (BP 90/55); **fever** (39.3°C); **tachypnea.** PE: nuchal rigidity resolved; mental status improved.

Labs   CBC: mild **anemia**; normal leukocytes. Lytes: **hypokalemia. BUN and creatinine** moderately **elevated.**

INFECTIOUS DISEASE

case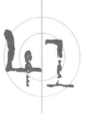

Amphotericin B Toxicity

Differential

Pneumonia

Sepsis

Discussion

The mechanism of action of amphotericin B is by **binding to ergosterol in fungi** and forming membrane pores. Toxicities include **arrhythmias, chills and fever, hypotension,** and **nephrotoxicity.**

Breakout Point

> The severe toxicity associated with amphotericin B, including chills and fever, have led to the term **SHAKE and BAKE.**

Treatment

If the reaction is severe, it may be necessary to lower the dosage of amphotericin B, use a liposomal form, or change to fluconazole. Pretreatment with antipyretics, antihistamines, and corticosteroids may lessen febrile symptoms.

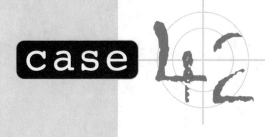

case 42

ID/CC	A 31-year-old truck driver visits a health clinic in San Diego complaining of **recurrent infections** (neutropenia), excessive **bleeding** (thrombocytopenia) and malaise, **weakness,** and apathy (anemia).
HPI	He travels south of the border daily and eats and sleeps there. He has had **typhoid fever** three times over the past 5 years, for which he has been treated with high-dose **powerful antibiotic.**
PE	VS: no fever; BP normal. PE: marked **pallor;** lungs clear; heart sounds normal; generalized **petechiae;** abdominal and neurologic examination unremarkable.
Labs	CBC: **anemia** (Hb 5.7); **leukopenia; thrombocytopenia.**
Imaging	CXR/KUB: within normal limits.
Micropathology	**Dry tap** seen on bone marrow biopsy with few hematopoetic precursors.

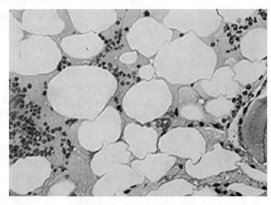

Figure 42-1. Note the abundance of fat. The few cellular elements are comprised primarily of lymphocytes

INFECTIOUS DISEASE

83

case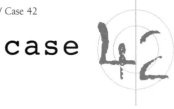

Chloramphenicol Side Effects

Differential

AIDS

Aplastic anemia

Agnogenic myeloid metaplasia

Myelophthisic anemia

Discussion

Chloramphenicol is a bacteriostatic antibiotic that acts by inhibiting peptidyl transferase in the **50S ribosomal unit.** It is active against anaerobes (abdominal sepsis) and rickettsiae as well as against typhoid fever and meningococcal, streptococcal, and *Haemophilus influenzae* meningitis. **Aplastic anemia** is nonetheless a major problem. Some aplastic cases appear to be related to overdose, while others are related to hypersensitivity to the drug. In infants, it produces the **gray-baby syndrome.** Owing to its potentially fatal side effect of **aplastic anemia,** chloramphenicol is used primarily for serious infections or acute *Salmonella typhi* infection.

Breakout Point

> Most bacteriostatic antibiotics interfere with protein production or metabolism within the bacteria. More frequently used bacteriostatic agents include:
> - Sulphonamides
> - Tetracyclines
> - Chloramphenicol
> - Erthryomycin
> - Trimethoprim

Treatment

Blood transfusions, antithymocyte globulin or cyclosporin, marrow transplantation.

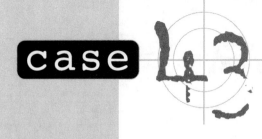

case 42

ID/CC   A 37-year-old missionary returning home from central **Africa** comes to the tropical medicine department of the local university for an evaluation of **blurred vision** and seeing "**halos**" **around lights** at night.

HPI   He also complains of marked **itching while showering** and notes that his **hair** has been turning prematurely **gray.** He has been taking **an antimalarial medication** for prophylaxis.

PE   "Half-moon-shaped" **corneal deposits** on funduscopic exam; diminished visual acuity bilaterally and **retinal edema** with pigmentation; slight **desquamation of palms of hands;** lungs clear; no heart murmurs; no hepatosplenomegaly; no focal neurologic signs.

Labs   CBC: moderate **leukopenia.**

Imaging   CXR: within normal limits.

case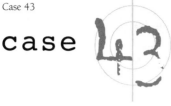

Chloroquine Toxicity

Differential

Multiple sclerosis

Glaucoma

Hypertensive retinopathy

Discussion

Chloroquine, a 4-aminoquinoline (acts by blocking DNA and RNA synthesis), is still one of the most widely used drugs for the **prophylaxis and treatment of malaria,** although resistant strains are becoming increasingly common. Its side effects include headache, dizziness, defects in lens accommodation with frontal heaviness, epigastralgia, diarrhea, and itching (primarily in dark-skinned people). It is also used to treat amebiasis, rheumatoid arthritis, and lupus erythematosus. When taken for long periods, it produces retinal edema with macular hyperpigmentation and chloroquine deposits with visual field defects as well as semicircular corneal opacities.

Treatment

Discontinue chloroquine or change to mefloquine as prophylaxis.

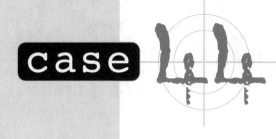

case

ID/CC A 25-year-old man presents with **spiking fevers, malaise, left-sided chest pain,** and **cough.**

HPI His symptoms started 2 weeks ago and have progressively worsened despite a full course of oral antibiotics. He also reports a history of prior **IV drug abuse.**

PE VS: fever (39.2°C); **tachycardia** (HR 105); **tachypnea.** PE: "amphoric" breath sounds heard over left lower lobe; S1 and S2 normally heard without murmurs, gallops or rubs.

Labs CBC: **leukocytosis, predominantly neutrophilic.** Blood cultures negative; induced sputum cultures grew **methicillin-resistant *Staphylococcus aureus.***

Imaging XR, chest: 2- by 3-cm cavities in right upper lobe of lung with air–fluid level. CT, chest: confirmed a left lower lobe **lung abscess.**

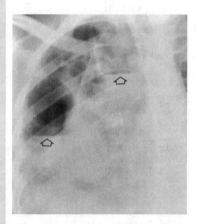

Figure 44-1. Multiple air–fluid levels (*arrow*) indicating abscess formation.

INFECTIOUS DISEASE

case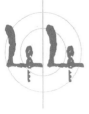

Drug Resistance

Differential
Pneumonia
Sepsis
Tuberculosis

Discussion
Antibiotic resistance is continuing to increase in both the hospital (nosocomial infections) and the community. Major resistant nosocomial organisms include *S. aureus*, **vancomycin-resistant enterococcus (VRE)**, *Klebsiella, Enterobacter, Escherichia coli, Pseudomonas,* and *Acinetobacter.* Multidrug-resistant bacteria causing community-acquired infections include **pneumococcus, gonococcus,** *Mycobacterium tuberculosis,* **group A streptococci, and** *E. coli.* Methicillin-resistant *S. aureus* (MRSA) is becoming widespread in a number of communities and is more commonly seen in **IV drug abusers, patients with recent hospitalizations,** and **residents in chronic care facilities.** Antibiotic resistance arises from numerous factors, including **colonization in hospital patients** and **frequent antibiotic use/abuse in the community.**

Breakout Point

In general, bacteria gain resistance to antibiotics by one of two general mechanisms:
1. Changes of bacterial permeability that alter the target of the anti-infectious agents
2. Synthesis of enzymes that inhibit the activity of the antibiotic

Treatment
Intravenous **vancomycin** therapy; add an **aminoglycoside** for synergistic bactericidal effect.

■ TABLE 44-1 MECHANISMS OF MICROBIAL DRUG RESISTANCE

Mechanism	Example: Antimicrobial	Example: Antineoplastic
Reduced Intracellular Concentration of Drug		
Inactive Drug	Inactivation of β-lactam antibiotics by β-lactamase	Inactivation of antimetabolites by deaminase
Prevent uptake of drug	Prevention of aminoglycoside entry by altered porins	Decreased methotrexate entry by decreased expression of reduced folate carrier
Promote efflux of drug	Efflux of multiple drugs by MDR membrane efflux pump	Efflux of multiple drugs by p170 membrane efflux pump
Altered Drug Target	Expression of altered peptidoglycan that no longer binds vancomycin	Expression of mutant DHFR that no longer binds methotrexate
Insensitivity to Apoptosis	N/A	Loss of active p53
Bypass Metabolic Requirement for Target	Inhibition of thymidylate synthase bypassed by exogenous thymidine	Loss of estrogen receptor-dependent growth results in tamoxifen resistance

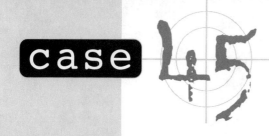

ID/CC   A 21-year-old college baseball player restarted his training 3 days ago, running 1,600 meters a day in preparation for the upcoming state tournament; yesterday he hit a home run and started off to first base when he suddenly fell to the ground and **could not walk** due to **acute pain** in the **Achilles tendon.**

HPI   He had recently spent 4 weeks in the hospital recovering from perforated appendicitis with peritonitis, where he received **IV antibiotic** for 2 weeks due to a surgical wound infection with *Pseudomonas aeruginosa* that was resistant to all other antibiotics.

PE   Surgical wound completely healed with no evidence of infection or postincisional hernia; Penrose drain orifice within normal limits; **inability to plantarflex left foot; Achilles tendon completely severed.**

Labs   CBC: no leukocytosis; no anemia. SMA-7 normal. UA: normal.

Imaging   CXR/KUB: within normal limits.

Micropathology   Achilles tendon shows inflammatory neutrophilic infiltrate with areas of hemorrhage and necrosis.

case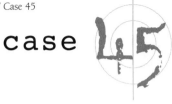

Fluoroquinolone Side Effects

Differential

Ankle sprain

Plantar fascitis

Tendon rupture

Discussion

Fluoroquinolones such as ciprofloxacin and nor-floxacin are bactericidal antibiotics that are active against **gram-negative rods**, including *Pseudomonas*; they are also active against *Neisseria* and some gram-positive organisms. They act by **inhibiting DNA gyrase** (TOPOISOMERASE II). Side effects include **damage to cartilage** (contraindicated in pregnancy and small children), tendonitis, and tendon rupture; they also produce gastric upset and nausea and may cause superinfections.

Breakout Point

Commonly used bactericidal antibiotics include:
• Penicillins
• Cephalosporins
• Vancomycin
• Aminoglycosides
• Fluoroquinolones
• Metronidazole

Treatment

Surgical repair.

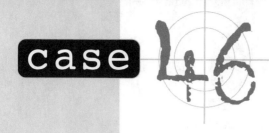

case 46

ID/CC   A 34-year-old woman presents with her family practitioner complaining of **hearing loss, vertigo**, and inability to walk properly due to **lack of balance**.

HPI   She is an otherwise healthy individual who underwent a left salpingectomy for pyosalpinx and was put on IV **antibiotic** for 10 days.

PE   Well hydrated, oriented, cooperative; gait is ataxic; abdomen shows well-healed, infraumbilical midline scar with no evidence of post-op hernia, infection, or hematoma.

Labs   **Elevated BUN** and **serum creatinine**; fractional excretion of sodium markedly increased ($>1\%$). UA: **dark brown granular casts** with free renal tubular epithelial cells and epithelial cell casts. ECG: normal sinus rhythm; no conduction abnormalities or signs of ischemia.

Imaging CXR: fails to disclose any lung infection or cardiac abnormality to account for the patient's symptoms.

case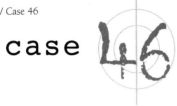

Gentamicin Side Effects

Differential

Ménière disease

Cerebellar stroke

Cyclophosphamide toxicity

Vancomycin toxicity

Discussion

Gentamicin is an **aminoglycoside** and thus shares the **ototoxicity** and **nephrotoxicity** of streptomycin, kanamycin, amikacin, and tobramycin. Ototoxicity is mainly cochlear and marked by ataxia and vertigo. Nephrotoxicity is minimized if care is taken to hydrate the patient and keep serum levels therapeutic. Transient elevations of BUN and creatinine are common.

Breakout Point

> Gentamicin as well as other aminoglycosides display **synergy when used with β-lactam antibiotics,** thus decreasing the dose of antibiotic required. Such synergy is used for serious enterococci infections.

Treatment

Supportive. Discontinuation of the aminoglycoside; resolution of acute episode may be delayed if patient remains hypovolemic, septic, or catabolic.

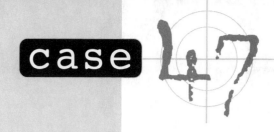

case 47

ID/CC A 23-year-old marathon runner visits his sports-medicine doctor complaining of unsightly, embarrassing **growth of his right breast** (GYNECOMASTIA) as well as **undue fatigue** after training and a slight yellowish hue in his eyes (JAUNDICE).

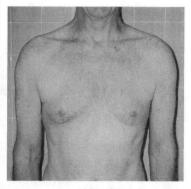

Figure 47-1. Gynecomastia.

HPI Three months ago, he was put on a daily oral **antifungal medication** because he had been suffering from a severe, refractory tinea corporis infection.

PE VS: bradycardia; **fever** (38.1°C). PE: slight jaundice in conjunctiva; no lymphadenopathy; no neck masses; cardiopulmonary exam normal; no hepatomegaly; examination of skin reveals tinea corporis covering intertriginous areas, buttocks, and scrotum.

Labs **AST and ALT increased**; serum bilirubin level increased.

Imaging US, liver: mildly enlarged liver.

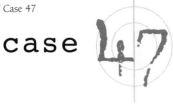

case 47

Ketoconazole Side Effects

Differential

Pituitary tumor

Anabolic steroid use

Weight gain

Discussion

Ketoconazole is an imidazole that inhibits fungal synthesis of ergosterol in membranes. It is used for blastomycosis, coccidioidomycosis, histoplasmosis, and candidiasis. Major side effects are **hepatic damage, gynecomastia, impotence** (due to inhibition of testosterone synthesis), inhibition of cytochrome P450, fever, and chills. When taken with antacids or H_2-receptor blockers, its absorption is decreased. It dramatically increases cyclosporine levels.

Breakout Point

> Although many drugs inhibit the hepatic P450 system, the more commonly mentioned drugs include:
> • Cimetidine
> • Ketoconazole
> • Erythromycin

Treatment

Discontinue drug; substitute treatment with alternative antifungal (e.g., terbinafine).

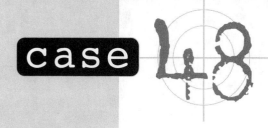

case 48

ID/CC A 21-year-old man comes to the health clinic because of the development of **fever,** marked **itching** all over his body, a **generalized urticarial rash** with **joint swelling,** and **difficulty breathing.**

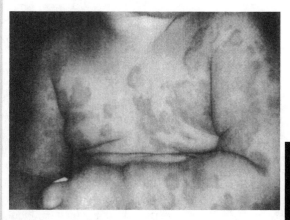

Figure 48-1. Urticarial rash.

HPI He just returned from a trip abroad, where he had developed a **purulent urethral discharge** (gonococcal urethritis) and went to a local doctor, who gave him "two shots on each side" preceded by two pills.

PE VS: mild **hypotension.** PE: in acute distress; mild cyanosis and difficulty breathing; eyelids, lips, and tongue **edematous;** large **hives** on hands and chest.

Labs CBC: leukocytosis (12,000 with 60% neutrophils). Lytes: normal.

Imaging CXR: normal.

case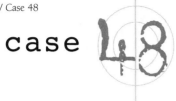

Penicillin Allergic Reaction

Differential

Angioedema

Mastocytosis

Vasovagal reaction

Red man syndrome

Discussion

Penicillins are antimicrobial drugs that block cell wall synthesis by inhibiting peptidoglycan cross-linking; they are bactericidal for gram-positive cocci and rods, gram-negative cocci, and spirochetes such as *Treponema pallidum*. Most adverse reactions to penicillin are allergic reactions that result when one of its metabolites acts as a hapten. Anaphylactic (TYPE I HYPERSENSITIVITY) reaction involves antigen reacting with IgE on presensitized mast cells and basophils; it is usually severe and immediate. Penicillin may also give rise to a **serum sickness** (TYPE III HYPERSENSITIV- ITY) reaction, an immune complex disorder with a lag period during which antibodies are formed. This results in fever, edema, malaise, arthralgias, and arthritis.

Breakout Point

> The incidence of cephalosporin allergy in patients with penicillin allergy is approximately 15%.

Treatment

Subcutaneous epinephrine, oxygen, hydrocortisone, antihistamines. Maintain airway and provide assisted ventilation if necessary. Severe reactions may result in laryngeal obstruction, hypotension, and death.

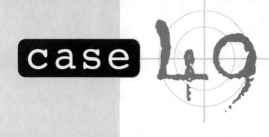

case 49

ID/CC	A 19-year-old military recruit comes to his medical officer complaining of **red urine** and **orange-colored staining of his T-shirt;** he also complains that every time he takes a **prophylactic antibiotic** for prevention of meningitis, he feels as if he has the flu (flulike response).
HPI	He underwent a routine physical exam and laboratory tests prior to joining the military camp and was started on the above medication at that time (meningococcus was found in nasopharyngeal secretions, indicating a meningococcal carrier state).
PE	VS: normal. PE: muscular male in no acute distress; no jaundice, hepatomegaly, spider angiomas, or parotid enlargement; nonpruritic maculopapular **rash** on chest and **petechial hemorrhages** on limbs.
Labs	**AST and ALT** moderately **increased.** UA: **proteinuria.** CBC: **thrombocytopenia.**
Imaging	CXR/KUB: normal.

case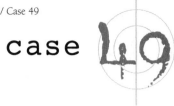

Rifampin Side Effects

Differential

Nephrolithiasis

Hepatitis

Thrombocytopenia

Influenza

Discussion

Rifampin is an antituberculous drug that acts by **inhibiting DNA-dependent RNA polymerase.** One of its major drawbacks is the rapid development of resistance if used alone. Other side effects include **discoloration of urine and sweat** with a yellowish-orange hue, **hepatic damage, skin rash, thrombocytopenia, tubulointerstitial nephritis,** and increased metabolism of anticoagulants and HIV protease inhibitors.

Breakout Point

> Rifampin is rarely used as a single agent in the treatment of any disease. It is, however, used as a single agent for prophylaxis. It is also important as a multidrug regiment for tuberculosis.

Treatment

Switch to ceftriaxone or ciprofloxacin for eradication of meningococcal carrier state.

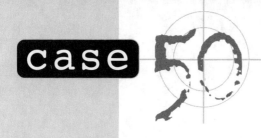

case 50

ID/CC A 9-year-old girl is seen in the ER for **vomiting.**

HPI Two days prior to admission she developed fever, chills, headache, myalgias, generalized fatigue, and cough. She was taken by her parents to a pediatrician yesterday and given **an antiviral medication** liquid suspension for the treatment of flu. After taking the first dose, she began to experience nausea that progressed to vomiting.

PE VS: **fever** (39.0°C); **tachycardia** (HR 110). PE: normal.

Labs CBC: leukocytosis.

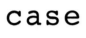

case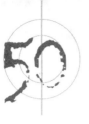

Tamiflu Therapy

Differential

Gastroenteritis

Food poisoning

Discussion

Oseltamivir is used for the treatment of **influenza types A and B** in adults and children; it decreases the duration and severity of flu symptoms if taken within 24 to 48 hours after symptoms begin. Along with **zanamivir**, it comprises a class of antiviral drugs called **neuroaminidase inhibitors**, which block the release of progeny viruses from infected cells. The most common adverse effect of oseltamivir is **vomiting**, which generally occurs only once and improves with continued dosing. Other events reported include **abdominal pain, epistaxis**, and **conjunctivitis**. Zanamivir can worsen pulmonary symptoms by decreasing peak expiratory flow rates in patients with underlying asthma or COPD.

Treatment

Symptomatic and supportive treatment; continue to administer Tamiflu and monitor for improvement in flu symptoms; discontinue use if vomiting persists despite use of antiemetics.

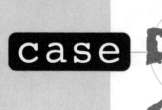
ID/CC   A 12-year-old **red-haired** girl visits her dermatologist at a local clinic because of a **rash** that appeared after she spent the **sunny** weekend hiking without sun block protection.

HPI   Two months ago, her dermatologist put her on low-dose **antibiotic** to prevent acne flare-ups.

PE   VS: normal. PE: patient **blue-eyed** and **fair-skinned**; red, nonpruritic, **maculopapular rash** that blanches on pressure on "V" of the anterior neck, posterior neck, forearms, hands, and face, sparing rest of body (rash is on sun-exposed areas of body); chest, abdomen, and neurologic exams fail to disclose pathology. **Brownish discoloration of the teeth.**

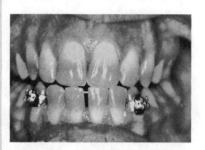

Figure 51-1. Staining of the teeth.

Labs   CBC/Lytes: normal. LFTs within normal limits. UA: mild **proteinuria**.

INFECTIOUS DISEASE

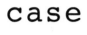

case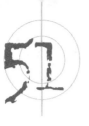

Tetracycline Side Effects

Differential

Sunburn

Allergic dermatitis

Discussion

Tetracyclines are **bacteriostatic antibiotics** that bind to the **30S ribosomal unit,** blocking synthesis of protein by preventing attachment of aminoacyl-tRNA. If they are taken with alkaline foods such as milk and antacids, GI absorption is decreased. Tetracycline is used both therapeutically and prophylactically for chlamydial genitourinary infections, Lyme disease, tularemia, cholera, and acne. Other side effects include **brownish discoloration of the teeth in children** (contraindicated in pregnancy), **photosensitivity,** aminoaciduria, proteinuria, phosphaturia, acidosis, and glycosuria (a Fanconi-like syndrome associated with "expired" tetracycline).

Breakout Point

Drugs that often cause photosensitivity:
- Tetracycline
- Amiodarone
- Sulfonamide
- Synthetic retinoids

Treatment

Sun protection, both mechanical and pharmacologic, while taking tetracycline.

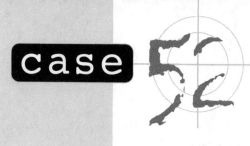

case 52

ID/CC An asymptomatic **HIV-positive** 29-year-old man visits his infectious disease specialist for a routine checkup; after determining his **CD4 count** (410), the physician decides to start him on oral **antiretroviral medication.**

HPI Two months later, he returns to the doctor's office feeling very **tired** (due to anemia); he has also had two **URIs,** and yesterday started **bleeding from his gums** (due to thrombocytopenia).

PE VS: slight tachycardia. PE: marked **pallor; disseminated petechiae** on arms and legs.

Labs CBC: **decreased platelets** (THROMBOCYTOPENIA); **decreased WBCs** (NEUTROPENIA); **decreased RBCs** (ANEMIA).

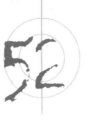

case 52

Zidovudine Toxicity

Differential

Worsening of underlying disease despite therapy

Blood loss anemia

Leukemia

Aplastic anemia

Discussion

AZT is a nucleoside analog antiretroviral agent that acts by inhibiting viral DNA chain elongation. It is used alone or in combination with other nucleoside analogs for the treatment of symptomatic or asymptomatic HIV infections. To prevent resistance, a protease inhibitor is also added to the regimen. Common side effects include anorexia, nausea, vomiting, fatigue, and insomnia. Nail hyperpigmentation, myopathy, lactic acidosis, and hepatic toxicity may also result from chronic AZT therapy.

Breakout Point

> Zidovudine (AZT) is approved for the prevention of perinatal infection in pregnant women with HIV, cutting the risk of transmission from mother the baby by nearly 70%.

Treatment

Consider adding erythropoieitin or switch to an alternative antiviral such as zalcitabine.

ID/CC A 59-year-old woman visits her family doctor complaining of **chronic fatigue**, **muscle weakness**, and **cramps**.

HPI She has been receiving **a diuretic medication** for the treatment of essential hypertension for more than 1 year.

PE VS: **tachycardia**. PE: **dehydration;** somnolence; muscle weakness; deep tendon reflexes slow.

Labs Elevated uric acid. Lytes: **decreased potassium and magnesium.** ECG: flattened T-waves and prominent U-waves (due to hypokalemia).

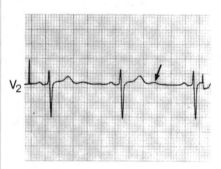

Figure 53-1. Prominent U Wave (Arrow).

case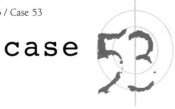

Loop Diuretic Side Effects

Differential

Anemia

Dehydration

Hyperaldosteronism

Discussion

Significant dehydration and electrolyte imbalance may occur in loop diuretic overdose. These compounds (**furosemide, bumetanide,** and **ethacrynic acid**) are potent diuretics that inhibit the **Na/K/2Cl** transport system, which can result in **hypokalemic metabolic alkalosis.** Potassium replacement and correction of hypovolemia can reverse this toxicity. Additional adverse effects include **ototoxicity, hyperuricemia, allergic reactions** (except for ethacrynic acid, which is not sulfa-derived), and **hypomagnesemia.**

Treatment

Treatment consists of replacement of fluid and electrolyte losses. Monitor ECG for cardiac abnormalities.

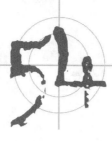

case 54

ID/CC A 76-year-old woman comes to her family doctor complaining of **constipation** and epigastric pain as well as **weakness** and painful **muscle cramps** (due to hypokalemia).

HPI She has a history of hypertension, for which she has been taking propranolol and **a diuretic medication** for the past several months.

PE VS: mild hypertension (BP 145/90); no fever. PE: well hydrated; funduscopic exam shows hypertensive retinopathy grade II; no increase in JVP; no masses in neck; no carotid bruit; soft S3 heard; no hepatomegaly; no pitting edema of lower legs; **deep tendon reflexes hypoactive** (due to hypokalemia).

Labs Hyperglycemia; increased BUN. Lytes: **hypokalemia; hyponatremia; hyperlipidemia; hyperuricemia; hypomagnesemia; hypercalcemia.** UA: proteinuria; high specific gravity. ABGs: **metabolic alkalosis.** ECG: S-T segment depression; broad, flat T-waves; U-waves (due to hypokalemia).

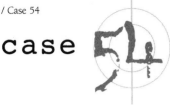

case 54

Thiazide Side Effects

Discussion

Thiazides, the most commonly used diuretics (of which hydrochlorothiazide is the prototype), are sulfonamide derivatives that act by **inhibiting sodium chloride reabsorption primarily in the early distal tubule.** They are used mainly in congestive heart failure, edematous states, and hypertension (they have a mild vasodilating effect). The hyperuricemia induced by thiazide diuretics can also precipitate bouts of **gout.**

Breakout Point

> Thiazide diuretics can often be associated with the development of SIADH.

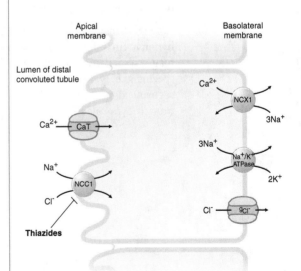

Figure 54-1. Mechanism of action of thiazides.

Treatment

Potassium-rich foods (chickpeas, bananas, papaya, citrus fruits, prunes), potassium supplement, or switch to potassium-sparing diuretics such as spironolactone and triamterene.

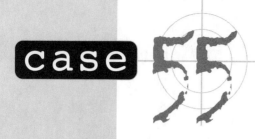

ID/CC A 48-year-old patient being treated for a large abscess in his lower back develops **oliguria**, **hematuria**, and an extensive **erythematous skin rash**.

HPI The patient has been treated according to culture and sensitivity of the pus from the abscess against *Staphylococcus aureus*. He has no history of allergy to any medications.

PE VS: fever (38.2°C); mild tachycardia. PE: erythematous **skin rash**; rales auscultated over left lung base.

Labs **Increased serum creatinine** and **BUN.** CBC: eosinophilia. Blood culture sterile. UA: mild **proteinuria; sterile pyuria;** urinary sediment shows abundant eosinophils and no bacteria.

Imaging US, abdomen: normal kidneys.

Micropathology Renal biopsy shows evidence of **tubulointerstitial disease**; inflammatory infiltrate in interstitium consists of a large number of eosinophils in addition to neutrophils, lymphocytes, and plasma cells.

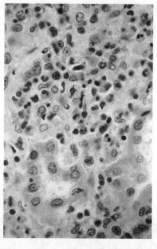

Figure 55-1. There is interstitial edema and infiltration by mononuclear leukocytes, with admixed eosinophils.

case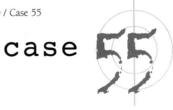

Tubulointerstitial Disease—Drug Induced

Differential	Allergic reaction
	Nephrolithiasis
	Acute renal failure
	Radiation nephritis
	Phenacetin use
Discussion	Drugs commonly associated with acute tubulointerstitial disease include **penicillin, ampicillin, thiazides, rifampin, methicillin,** and **cimetidine.** This type II hypersensitivity reaction is often reversed with cessation of offending drug; if it is not reversed, it may progress to renal failure.
Treatment	Alternative antibiotic therapy and supportive management; cessation of offending drug often reverses disease.

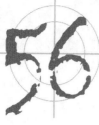

case 56

ID/CC A 50-year-old man presents with **flushed skin, headaches, upset stomach, photophobia,** and **blue-tinted vision.**

HPI He has been diagnosed with **erectile dysfunction** in the past and is currently on an appropriate medication. He has no history of **diabetes** or of **cardiovascular, prostate,** or **anxiety problems.** He also takes cimetidine regularly for acid reflux.

PE VS: **hypotension** (BP 90/50). PE: **plethoric** face; **nasal congestion.**

Labs CBC/Lytes: normal. LFTs normal. ECG: normal.

case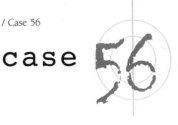

Viagra (Sildenafil) Therapy

Differential
Carcinoid syndrome
Niacin therapy
Red man syndrome

Discussion
Sildenafil, which acts by inhibiting phosphodi-esterase, enhances the effect of **nitric oxide,** an endogenous **vasodilator** that relaxes penile smooth muscle and allows blood to flow in, producing an erection. Side effects are dose-related. Sildenafil is **absolutely contraindicated** when **nitrates** are used for treatment of **angina** and should be used cautiously in patients taking **antihypertensive medications** or with preexisting cardiovascular disease. Reported deaths due to sildenafil are typically **cardiovascular events** in **elderly men** (65 or more years of age). Sildenafil is metabolized by the liver via the **cytochrome P450** system and should be used cautiously in patients taking cimetidine, erythromycin, rifampin, and ketoconazole.

Treatment
Adjust medications as necessary to prevent **cytochrome P450 interactions** with sildenafil. In this case, switch the patient from cimetidine to another H_2-receptor–blocking agent with fewer interactions (such as ranitidine).

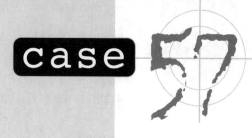

case 57

ID/CC   A 28-year-old woman is started on **anti-flu prophy-laxis**; she teaches at a school where there has been an **influenza** outbreak.

HPI   One week later, she started feeling **dizzy** and having **problems walking normally** (ATAXIA). An ENT consult ruled out middle-ear causes of vertigo.

PE   VS: **no fever**; remainder of vital signs normal. PE: **speech** somewhat **slurred**; **gait ataxic**; no focal neurologic signs.

Labs   CBC/Lytes/UA: normal.

Imaging   MR/CT: no intracranial pathology.

case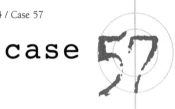

Amantadine Toxicity

Differential

Benign vertigo

Ménière disease

Labyrinthitis

Cerebellar dysfunction

Discussion

Amantadine is an antiviral agent that blocks viral penetration and uncoating. It also causes the release of dopamine from intact nerve terminals (sometimes used for treatment of **Parkinson disease**). It is used as **prophylaxis against influenza A.** Toxicity includes cerebellar problems such as **ataxic gait, slurred speech,** and **dizziness.** Elderly patients with renal insufficiency are more susceptible to toxicity.

Treatment

Discontinue amantadine. Amantadine is not effectively removed by dialysis because of its large volume of distribution.

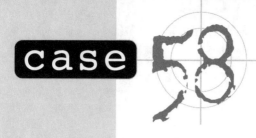
case 58

ID/CC A 24-year-old woman visits her physician because of **pain in her arm** after spending all day cleaning the basement of her house; x-rays taken as a routine procedure revealed a **linear fracture** of the right radius.

HPI She is an epileptic who has been treated for 3 years with **anti-seizure medication.** She states that she has been suffering from increasing **leg weakness** and persistent **lower back pain.**

PE VS: normal. PE: **increase in size of gums** (GINGIVAL HYPERPLASIA); no neck masses; **hirsutism** present; linear right radial fracture

Labs **Megaloblastic anemia;** BUN and creatinine normal; **glucose mildly elevated; increased alkaline phosphatase;** decreased levels of vitamin D; **hypocalcemia; hypophosphatemia.**

Imaging XR: right radial fracture; **shortening of lumbar vertebrae; generalized osteopenia and Looser lines** (MILKMAN FRACTURES; PATHOGNOMONIC). DEXA: confirms presence of severe osteopenia.

case

Anticonvulsant Osteomalacia

Differential

Osteoporosis

Steroid use

Collagen disorders

Discussion

Phenytoin and, to a lesser extent, other antiepileptic drugs such as phenobarbital and carbamazepine may cause **vitamin D deficiency** with consequent development of osteomalacia (in adults) and rickets (in children). Fractures with minor trauma may be a presenting sign, as may bone pain and proximal muscle weakness.

Breakout Point

> Phenytoin also inhibits folate absorption. That is, in part, why it is contraindicated during pregnancy, as folate is required to prevent neural tube defects.

Treatment

Switch to other antiepileptics; vitamin D and càlcium and folate supplements; bisphosphonate therapy; treat fracture, physiotherapy.

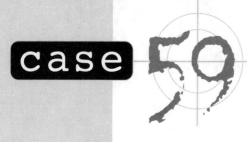

ID/CC A 45-year-old **woman** comes to her family physician for an evaluation of frequent URIs (due to neutropenia) and gum bleeding (due to thrombocytopenia). She also complains of **double vision** (DIPLOPIA), nausea, **sleepiness,** and **dry mouth** as well as difficulty walking.

HPI She has been suffering from recurrent, severe, sharp pain on the left side of her face that radiates to the corner of her eye and is triggered by mastication or cold exposure (TRIGEMINAL NEURALGIA). She has been taking an **antiepileptic medication** for several months, during which time her attacks have been much less frequent.

PE VS: normal. PE: well hydrated, oriented, and in no acute distress; **ataxic gait;** funduscopic exam normal except for mild **mydriasis.**

Labs CBC: **decreased platelets; decreased neutrophil count.** Coagulation and bleeding time increased. LP: CSF normal. No evidence of multiple sclerosis on evoked-potential testing; **AST and ALT** moderately **increased;** serum carbamazepine level supratherapeutic (>12 mg/dL).

Imaging CT, brain: normal.

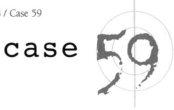

case

Carbamazepine Side Effects

Differential
Immune-suppressed state
Multiple sclerosis
Antipsychotic medication use

Discussion
Trigeminal neuralgia is sometimes seen in association with multiple sclerosis, primarily in younger patients. Carbamazepine is chemically similar to imipramine and has been used for trigeminal neuralgia as well as for the treatment of partial and tonic-clonic seizures.

Treatment
Consider alternative treatment options for trigeminal neuralgia, such as baclofen, clonazepam, phenytoin, or valproic acid.

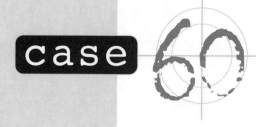

NEUROLOGY

ID/CC A pediatrician is called upon to evaluate a 5-week old infant with multiple birth defects.

HPI The mother is a 17-year-old runaway who was homeless, had no prenatal care, and continued her habit of **substance abuse throughout her pregnancy.**

PE **Small head size** (MICROCEPHALY); **facial flattening** with **epicanthal folds;** small eyes (MICROPHTHALMOS); **cardiac murmur** (diagnosed as an atrial septal defect); chest deformed (pectus excavatum).

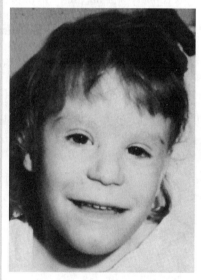

Figure 60-1. Characteristic facies as a child.

Labs CBC: mild anemia. Increased AST and ALT.

Imaging CXR: cardiomegaly; pectus excavatum deformity. XR, hip: congenital dislocation of left hip.

119

case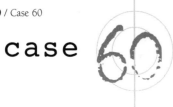

Fetal Alcohol Syndrome

Differential

Down syndrome

DiGeorge syndrome

Neglect

Inborn error in metabolism

Discussion

Alcohol is the leading cause of fetal malformations in the United States. Fetal alcohol syndrome may cause myriad abnormalities, both skeletal and visceral, but usually involves a triad of features: (1) craniofacial dysmorphology, including mild to moderate **microcephaly** and **maxillary hypoplasia;** (2) prenatal and postnatal **growth retardation;** and (3) CNS abnormalities, including **mental retardation,** with IQs often in the range of 50 to 70. In addition, fetal alcohol exposure leads to an increased incidence of **cardiac malformations,** including **patent ductus arteriosus** and **septal defects.** Risk is dose related.

Treatment

No specific treatment available; treat each malformation/disease accordingly.

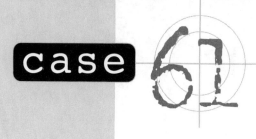

ID/CC   A 23-year-old woman is terrified after reportedly seeing grotesque monsters trying to kill her while she had her left **dislocated shoulder** reduced.

HPI   She injured her shoulder while rock-climbing in Colorado. The doctor was called upon to see her immediately after the accident. She did not suffer major injuries but had a dislocated shoulder and was not cooperative enough to tolerate the procedure (reduction) without medication, so he anesthetized her with **a dissociative anesthetic**, atropine, and diazepam.

Imaging   X-rays at time of injury showed an anterior shoulder dislocation.

case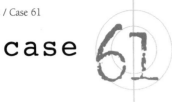

Ketamine Side Effects

Differential

Psychosis

Bipolar disorder

Peyote use

LSD use

Discussion

Ketamine is an arylcyclohexylamine that produces a **dissociative anesthesia;** the patient has open eyes, and muscle tone is preserved (with sufficient analgesia to do major surgery and total amnesia). Its major side effect is **vivid hallucinations,** sometimes terrifying, upon arousal, mostly in adults. It is widely used in developing countries, in rural areas where there is no available anesthesiologist, and in short pediatric procedures (abscess debridement, burn wounds, dressing changes, etc.) because of its relative safety and lack of life-threatening side effects (such as respiratory depression, which is common with other anesthetics). However, it also causes cardiac stimulation with increased blood pressure and tachycardia.

Treatment

Benzodiazepines (e.g., diazepam) reduce the adverse effects of ketamine.

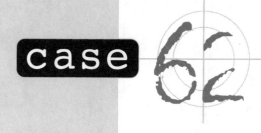

case

ID/CC An 82-year-old man complains to his doctor about chronic **nausea** and vomiting, **loss of appetite**, and **altered taste perception** as well as **involuntary tremors, chewing, and grimacing movements** (DYSKINESIA).

HPI The patient also states he has been having **palpitations** and **insomnia.** He suffers from Parkinson disease and has been taking **appropriate medications** for a long time.

PE VS: **tachycardia** (HR 115); **postural hypotension.** PE: patient thin; typical parkinsonian gait; masklike facies; pill-rolling tremor of hands; **choreiform movements** of head and hands; grimacing facial movements.

Labs CBC/PBS: **Coombs test positive;** no hemolytic anemia. ECG: **premature ventricular contractions** (cause of palpitations). Urine and saliva are brownish in color.

case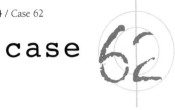

Levodopa Side Effects

Differential | Worsening of Parkinson disease
Gastroenteritis

Discussion | Dopamine cannot cross the blood–brain barrier; however, levodopa, a precursor of dopamine, does. When this drug is administered, it is usually given in combination with carbidopa, an inhibitor of the peripheral dopa decarboxylase (thus increasing the half-life and plasma levels of levodopa). **Dyskinesias** are a common side effect, as are **GI symptoms** (nausea and vomiting) and postural hypotension. Arrhythmias, anxiety, depression, insomnia, and confusion have also been reported. The dose of levodopa must be slowly decreased, because **abrupt cessation** may result in an **akinetic state.** Many patients eventually experience a decline in efficacy with levodopa/carbidopa. They may develop an "on-off" phenomenon in which they suddenly lose activity of the levodopa and are "frozen." Other patients experience a more gradual decline in which the levodopa effect lasts for shorter periods of time.

Treatment | Minimize side effects by taking drug with meals or in smaller doses. Often, administration of carbidopa diminishes side effects. Tolerance to emetic effect may also develop. Antiemetics may be given, but these may reduce antiparkinsonian effects.

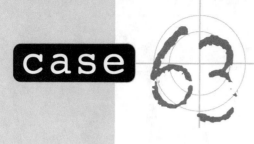

ID/CC A 16-year-old woman undergoes **surgery** to remove an inflamed appendix and has a **rare anesthesia complication**.

HPI The father states that the patient's paternal uncle died of an anesthetic complication. The patient has had no prior surgery and received general anesthesia.

PE VS: very high **fever** (39.8°C); **hypertension** (BP 150/95). PE: generalized **muscular rigidity** with difficulty breathing, anxiety, and marked sweating.

Labs CBC: leukocytosis with neutrophilia. Lytes: **hyperkalemia**. ABGs: metabolic acidosis. **Elevated CK.**

case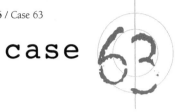

Malignant Hyperthermia

Differential | Heat stroke
Thalamic injury
Status epilepticus
Lethal catatonia

Discussion | Malignant hyperthermia is a highly lethal, genetically determined **myopathy (autosomal-dominant** trait). It is triggered by **inhalation anesthetics** (more commonly halothane), particularly those coupled with succinylcholine. The syndrome includes **tachycardia, hypertension, acidosis, hyperkalemia,** and **muscle rigidity,** and it appears to be related to excess myoplasmic calcium.

Breakout Point

> Some patients with maligant hyperthermia have mutations in the sarcoplasmic reticulum ryanodine receptor.

Treatment | Immediate treatment to lower body temperature, control acidosis, and restore electrolyte balance is critical to survival. **IV dantrolene** relaxes skeletal muscle by inhibiting release of calcium from sarcoplasmic reticulum. This allows muscle to relax and limits hyperthermia from muscle hyperactivity.

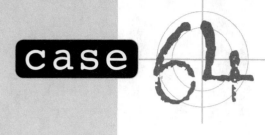

case 64

ID/CC   A 32-year-old man is brought by his wife to the family care center of the community because of increasing **tremors, slowing of movements** (BRADYKINESIA), and **postural instability.**

HPI   The patient works as a **chemist** at a leading pharmaceutical research company in Northern California and has a long-standing history of **drug abuse requiring hospitalization.**

PE   VS: normal. PE: flat facies; **resting tremor; cogwheel rigidity;** impaired capacity for voluntary motor activity; speech slow, as are voluntary movements.

Imaging   CT, head: no apparent intracranial pathology.

case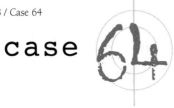

Parkinson Disease—MPTP-Induced

Differential

Seizures

Transient ischemic attack

Closed head injury

Tardive dyskinesia

Discussion

Several drugs may produce Parkinson-like symptoms, including haloperidol and phenothiazines, which block dopamine receptors, as well as reserpine and tetrabenazine, which deplete biogenic monoamines from their storage sites. In their attempts to produce "designer drugs" related to meperidine, "underground" chemists have also synthesized a compound, 1-methyl-4-phenyl-tetrahydrobiopteridine (MPTP). The toxicity of MPTP is produced by its oxidation to **MPP+** (a toxic compound), which selectively **destroys the dopaminergic neurons in the substantia nigra.**

Treatment

No effective therapy currently exists for treatment of drug-induced Parkinson syndrome aside from discontinuation of offending drug.

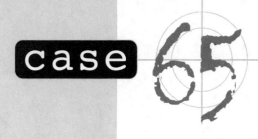

case 65

ID/CC   A 21-year-old man who emigrated to the United States 3 months ago visits a neighborhood medical clinic complaining of apprehension, tremors, **dizziness, inability to walk properly, and double vision** (DIPLOPIA).

HPI   He is a newly diagnosed epileptic whose understanding of English is very poor, so when his doctor prescribed one tablet of **anti-seizure medication** every 24 hours, he thought the doctor meant one tablet every 2 to 4 hours.

PE   VS: hypotension; bradycardia. PE: bilateral nystagmus with sluggish pupils; patient is slightly lethargic; ataxic gait; dysarthria.

Labs   CBC: megaloblastic anemia. Moderate increases in AST and ALT. ECG: sinus bradycardia. Serum phenytoin level supratherapeutic.

Imaging   CXR: normal. CT, head: no intracranial pathology seen.

case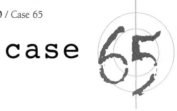

Phenytoin Overdose

Differential

Multiple sclerosis

Cerebellar dysfunction

Discussion

Overdose **may be lethal** owing to the ability of phenytoin to induce CNS, cardiac, and respiratory depression. Certain drugs, such as INH, cimetidine, and sulfonamides, can increase phenytoin levels by inhibiting the microsome enzymes that are responsible for the metabolism of phenytoin. The rate of hydroxylation of phenytoin also varies among individuals as a result of genetic differences.

Treatment

Gastric lavage or activated charcoal if acute overdose. Stop treatment temporarily; then resume at proper dosage.

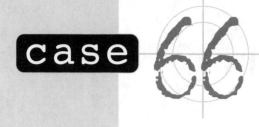
ID/CC   A 65-year-old woman with long-standing **osteoarthritis** presents with **bilateral lower-extremity swelling**.

HPI   For the last 2 months, she has been taking **an anti-inflammatory medication** for relief of joint pain and inflammation.

PE   VS: normal. PE: JVP normal; S1 and S2 auscultated normally without any murmurs, gallops, or rubs; **mild, bilateral pitting lower extremity edema**.

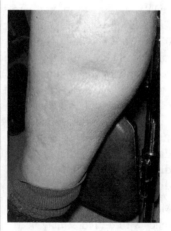

Figure 66-1. Lower extremity pitting edema.

Labs   CBC/Lytes: normal. LFTs normal. ECG: normal.

case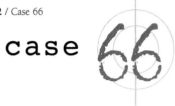

Cox-II Inhibitors

Differential

Lymphedema

Congestive heart failure

Deep vein thrombosis

Discussion

Celecoxib is a nonsteroidal anti-inflammatory drug (NSAID) used to treat **osteoarthritis** and adult **rheumatoid arthritis.** Recently, it has also been used to reduce the number of **colorectal polyps** in patients with **familial adenomatous polyposis (FAP)** and shows promise in treating GI cancers. Celecoxib works by inhibiting **cyclooxygenase-2 (COX-2),** but unlike other NSAIDs, it does not inhibit COX-1. As a result, there is a postulated **reduction in the incidence of upper GI ulcers** as compared to aspirin, ibuprofen, and naproxen, as well as less interference with blood platelets/clotting. Celecoxib is contraindicated in patients who are allergic to sulfa drugs or aspirin. It can also cause **liver damage** and/or **edema.** The **efficacy** of **thiazide diuretics, loop diuretics, and ACE inhibitors** is **diminished** by celecoxib.

Treatment

Monitor for worsening edema; provide temporary relief with diuretics; may need to switch to an alternative NSAID.

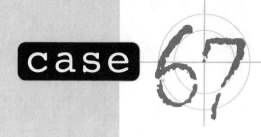

ID/CC	An 18-year-old high-school dropout is brought to the ER because of marked **restlessness, euphoria, anxiety, tachycardia, paranoia,** and **agitation.**
HPI	The patient is a known **drug abuser** with an otherwise unremarkable medical history.
PE	VS: marked **hypertension** (BP 185/100); **tachycardia** (HR 165). PE: **diaphoresis; tremor.**
Labs	UA: **occult hemoglobin** (due to **rhabdomyolysis** with **myoglobinuria**).

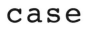 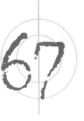

Amphetamine Abuse

Differential
Hypertensive emergency
Hyperthyroidism
Anticholinergic toxicity
Theophylline toxicity
Panic attack

Discussion
A variety of amphetamines are used clinically, including methylphenidate (Ritalin) for attention deficit hyperactivity disorder (ADHD). However, many of these drugs are commonly abused as well. Such agents activate CNS via peripheral release of catecholamines, inhibition of reuptake mechanisms, or inhibition of monoamine oxidase enzymes. Excretion is dependent on urine pH, with optimal excretion occurring in acidified urine.

Breakout Point

> Recently the **first nonstimulant drug for the treatment of ADHD,** Atomoxetine, was approved. This drug is a selective norepinephrine reuptake inhibitor.

Treatment
Treat agitation, seizures, and coma if they occur; treat hypertension with benzodiazepines; if refractory or severe, use IV vasodilators such as phentolamine or nitroprusside. Propranolol is used to prevent tachyarrhythmias.

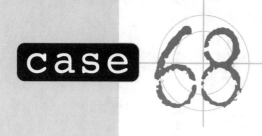

case 68

ID/CC A 20-year-old medical student is brought to the emergency room because his roommate noticed that he had been **sleeping all day** and awakening from time to time with **nightmares;** the patient then stated that **he wanted to shoot himself** and began to look for a gun.

HPI He had just finished end-of-year exams in all his subjects, for which he had studied late into the night and had taken **a stimulant** daily for several weeks.

PE VS: mild tachycardia. PE: well-oriented with respect to time, person, and place but very **lethargic** and complains of a severe **headache;** funduscopic exam normal; no increased JVP; no neck masses; lungs clear; heart sounds with no murmurs; abdomen soft and nontender with no masses; peristaltic sounds increased (patient complains of abdominal cramps when these are heard).

Labs Routine lab exams fail to disclose abnormality.

Imaging CXR: no cardiopulmonary pathology apparent.

case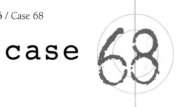

Amphetamine Withdrawal

Differential | Depression
Hypothyroidism
Cocaine withdrawal
Caffeine withdrawal

Discussion | Amphetamines are used recreationally for their ability to produce a sense of well-being and euphoria, with sympathetic stimulation. There are also some medical indications for their use, such as hyperactivity. Amphetamines may be abused orally or parenterally or may be smoked. **Withdrawal symptoms** include lethargy, **suicidal thoughts, profound depression,** intestinal colic, headache, sleepiness, and nightmares.

Treatment | Hospitalization due to risk of suicide, antidepressants, supportive treatment.

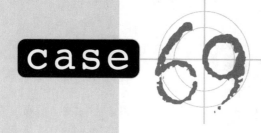

case 69

ID/CC	A 19-year-old **epileptic** student is brought by ambulance to the emergency room in a **coma** after being found on the floor of her apartment.
HPI	She had been feeling depressed for several months and, according to her roommate, had just broken up with her boyfriend. She took a **whole bottle of her antiepileptic pills** at once.
PE	She was brought to the ER **unconscious, hypotensive, hypothermic** (35°C), and **bradypneic.** PE: no response to verbal stimulation; reacts only to painful stimuli; **bullae** on lower legs; deep tendon **reflexes slow** (HYPOREFLEXIA).
Labs	ABGs: pronounced **hypoxemia** and **respiratory acidosis. Blood alcohol level also increased.** ECG: sinus bradycardia.
Imaging	CXR: no evidence of aspiration (a common complication of sedative overdose due to diminished gag reflex and altered consciousness).
Gross Pathology	**Globus pallidus necrosis** with pulmonary and cerebral edema.

case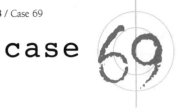

Barbiturate Intoxication

Differential

Post-ictal state

Hypoglycemia

Encephalitis

Carbon monoxide poisoning

Gamma-hydroxybutyrate use (date rape drug)

Discussion

Barbiturates facilitate GABA action by increasing the duration of the chloride channel opening; they are used as antianxiety drugs, in sleep disorders, and in anesthesia. Barbiturates **induce the cytochrome P450 system** of liver microsomal enzymes, thereby affecting the metabolism of several drugs. In overdose, death may ensue due to severe **respiratory depression** or **aspiration pneumonia**.

Treatment

Airway maintenance; oxygen; assisted ventilation; gastric lavage; cathartics; alkalinization of urine; warming blankets; consider pressors, hemodialysis or hemoperfusion. **Flumazenil reverses benzodiazepine overdose but not barbiturate overdose.**

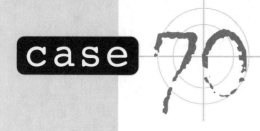

ID/CC A 14-year old boy is brought to the ER by his anxious mother for **mild somnolence, mild stupor,** and **mild motor dysfunction.** The patient initially answers negatively to questions about drug use.

HPI Upon further private questioning, he reveals that he had been using an **illicit substance.**

PE VS: tachycardia; mild tachypnea. PE: **conjunctiva red** and injected.

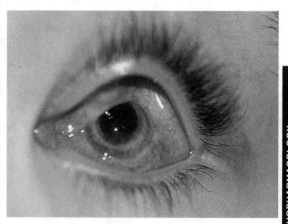

Figure 70-1. Conjunctival injection.

Labs UA: presence of **drugs of abuse.**

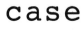 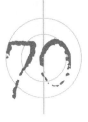

Cannabis Intoxication

Differential

Overall fatigue

Depression

Hallucinogen use

Schizophrenia

Alcoholism

Discussion

The primary psychoactive agent in marijuana is delta-9-tetrahydro-cannabinol, which is released during pyrolysis (smoking) of *Cannabis sativa*. Acute cannabis intoxication usually consists of a **subjective perception of relaxation** and **mild euphoria** accompanied by **mild impairment in thinking, concentration,** and **perceptual** and **psychosocial functions.** Chronic abusers may lose interest in common socially desirable goals. **Therapeutic effects include treatment for glaucoma, prevention of emesis** associated with cancer chemotherapy, and **appetite stimulation** ("THE MUNCHIES").

Treatment

No specific therapy; reassurance; benzodiazepines as needed for anxiety.

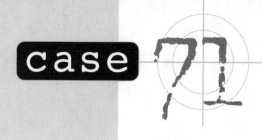

case 72

ID/CC A 24-year-old woman of Ashkenazi Jewish background complains to her family doctor of **repeated URIs** (due to neutropenia), increasing **fatigue, muscle aches,** and **headaches.**

HPI She had been showing flattening of affect, suspiciousness, a delusional mood, and auditory hallucinations that were diagnosed as **schizophrenia** 3 years ago. She was recently switched to a new medication because other antipsychotics were unsuccessful.

PE VS: **fever;** tachycardia (HR 165). PE: patient in obvious discomfort; **pallor** (due to anemia); conscious and oriented to person, place, and time; **petechiae** (due to thrombocytopenia) on chest and arms; cardiopulmonary, abdominal, and genital exams normal; no extrapyramidal signs.

Labs CBC: agranulocytosis.

Imaging CXR: No signs of lung infection.

case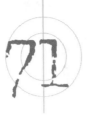

Clozapine Toxicity

Differential

Anemia

Influenza

Parvovirus infection

Leukemia

Discussion

Clozapine is used for the treatment of schizophrenia and psychotic disorders that are unresponsive to other therapy. It blocks D_1, D_2, and D_4 dopamine receptors as well as serotonin receptors. Because of its **low affinity for D_2 receptors,** clozapine causes few extrapyramidal symptoms. Agranulocytosis occurs in <2% of patients, but all patients must receive weekly blood counts to monitor for this potentially lethal effect. Other side effects include seizures, sedation, and anticholinergic symptoms. Agranulocytosis usually reverses with discontinuation of clozapine.

Treatment

Discontinue clozapine and institute alternate pharmacotherapy; granulocyte colony-stimulating factor in severe cases.

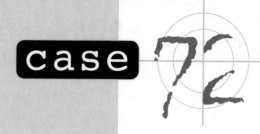

case 72

ID/CC   A 32-year-old stockbroker is brought to the ER after police find him **hiding in an alley.**

HPI   The patient had been at a **party** with several friends. He admits to indulging in an **illicit drug** from a new dealer for the past 6 hours. He complains of some chest pain

PE   VS: **hypertension** (BP 180/95); **tachycardia** (HR 160). PE: **restless, malnourished,** and **disoriented.** EKG: Sinus tachycardia and **ST elevation** in inferior and precordial leads.

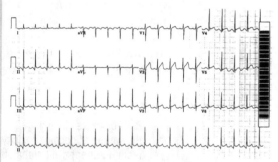

Figure 72-1. Sinus tachycardia with ST elevation is present in both inferior and precordial leads.

case 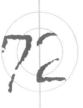72

Cocaine Abuse

Differential

Psychotic state
Paranoid state
Malignant hypertension
Hyperthyroidism
Amphetamine use

Discussion

Cocaine is a CNS stimulant and an inhibitor of neuronal catecholamine reuptake mechanisms; hence, its use results in a state of generalized sympathetic stimulation, with typical symptoms including **euphoria, anxiety, psychosis,** and **hyperactivity.** Severe **hypertension, ventricular tachycardia,** or **fibrillation** may also occur. **Angina pectoris** in a young, healthy person is suggestive of cocaine use. **Myocardial infarction** secondary to **coronary vasospasm** and thrombosis have been described as well.

Breakout Point

> Beta-blockers, in general, are best avoided in the setting of cocaine toxicity because they may result in unopposed alpha effects of cocaine.

Treatment

Monitor vital signs and ECG for several hours. There are no specific antidotes for cocaine use. Control hypertension with benzodiazepines and **phentolamines;** avoid beta-blockers to prevent paradoxical hypertension (from unopposed alpha-vasoconstriction). In severe cases, treat dysrhythmias with IV sodium bicarbonate or lidocaine. Dialysis and hemoperfusion are not effective.

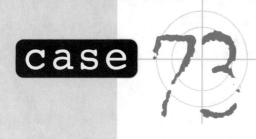

case 72

ID/CC A 36-year-old man, an ENT doctor, tells his psychiatrist that he has been feeling terribly **depressed** and **anxious** over the last 3 weeks.

HPI The patient has been in good health, but he recently entered into a **drug rehabilitation program** to **wean himself off a drug of abuse.**

PE VS: tachycardia; BP normal; no fever. PE: patient expresses concern over his increasing **lethargy, depression, hunger,** and **extreme cravings for stimulants.**

Labs Basic lab work and tox screen are all within normal limits. ECG: sinus tachycardia.

case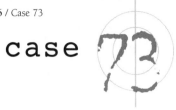

Cocaine Withdrawal

Differential | Depression
Generalized anxiety disorder
Amphetamine withdrawal

Discussion | Symptoms of cocaine withdrawal may be due to enhanced sensitivity of inhibitory receptors on dopaminergic neurons. In contrast to mild physiologic withdrawal signs and symptoms, cocaine produces **marked psychological dependency** and behavioral withdrawal symptoms.

Treatment | No definitive treatment exists to alleviate symptoms of cocaine withdrawal and associated cravings. Bromocriptine, a dopamine agonist that is used in Parkinson disease, has been reported to diminish cocaine cravings.

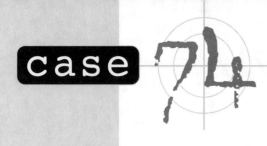case 74

ID/CC   A 35-year-old plastic **surgeon** is rushed to the hospital by his wife after he is found lying comatose in his bed with a couple of **syringes lying on the floor** and his sleeve rolled up.

HPI   His wife states that her husband had been having serious financial problems; she has suspected drug use in light of recent **personality and mood changes.**

PE   On admission to ER, patient had a tonic-clonic **seizure; respiratory depression;** bradycardia; stupor; **pupils very constricted** (PINPOINT PUPILS); cold skin; hypotension; marked hyporeflexia; hypoactive bowel sounds; **needle "train track" marks** (stigmata of multiple previous injections).

Labs   ABGs: hypoxemia; hypercapnia; respiratory acidosis.

Imaging   CXR: **noncardiogenic pulmonary edema** (edema without cardiomegaly).

Gross Pathology   Pulmonary congestion and edema; inflammatory neutrophilic infiltrate of arteries in brain and lung.

Micropathology   Brain cell swelling due to hypoxia.

case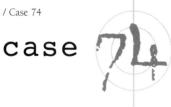

Heroin Overdose

Differential

Hypoglycemia

Diabetic ketoacidosis

Hypernatremia

Hypoxia

Closed head trauma

Salicylate toxicity

Discussion

Heroin is a synthetic derivative of morphine that is abused as a recreational drug. Health professionals have a higher incidence of opioid abuse, generally abusing medical opioids. Heroin abuse is a complex social disease that is linked with violence, prostitution, crime, antisocial behavior, and premature death; it may result in fatal overdose, endocarditis, fungal infections, abscess formation, anaphylaxis, and HIV transmission. Death may result from aspiration of gastric contents or from apnea.

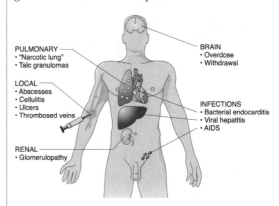

Figure 74-1. Complications of intravenous drug use.

Treatment

Establish a patent airway, assist ventilation, correct acid–base disorders, hypothermia, and hypotension. **Naloxone** as specific antagonist (naloxone may induce rapid opiate withdrawal), with follow-up in ICU.

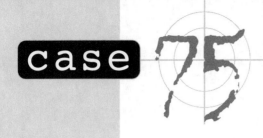

case 75

ID/CC   A 26-year-old woman who models for photography magazines is referred to the dermatologist by her family doctor because of **persistent acne** that has been unresponsive to the usual treatment.

HPI   She also complains of **constant thirst**, dryness of the mouth, and **frequent urination.** She has been diagnosed with **bipolar affective disorder** with **manic** predominance and was recently started on **a mood-stabilizing medication.**

PE   Sensorium normal; oriented and cooperative; fine resting tremor of hands; **mouth is dry;** no signs of present depression or mania; face shows presence of **severe cystic acne** on chin, forehead, and upper chest with **folliculitis;** mucous membranes dry.

Labs   CBC: **leukocytosis.** Lytes: mild hyponatremia. BUN and creatinine normal; pregnancy test negative. ECG: T-wave inversion.

case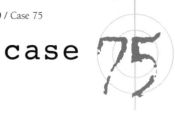

Lithium Side Effects

Differential

Diabetes mellitus
Hypothyroidism
Schizophrenia
Heavy metal toxicity

Discussion

Lithium is the preferred treatment for the manic stage of bipolar affective disorder; however, its mechanism of action on mood stability is still unclear. One possibility revolves around lithium's effects on the **IP$_3$ second-messenger system** in the brain. The onset of action may take several days, and side effects may be very bothersome, such as persistent **polyuria** and **polydipsia** (ADH antagonism), weight gain, and severe acne. It is contraindicated in pregnancy due to its teratogenic effect.

Breakout Point

> Lithium can also cause clinically apparent **hypothyroidism.** Patients must have their thyroid-stimulating hormones checked and synthetic thyroid hormone administered, if necessary.

Treatment

Decrease or discontinue lithium use; severe cases may need dialysis; treat acne with isotretinoin (teratogenic), tetracycline, or benzoyl peroxide.

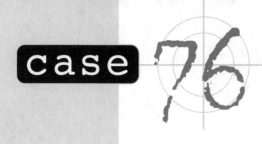

case 76

ID/CC	A 40-year-old man was brought into the ER by his sister, who reported that he had dropped by her apartment **acting "drunk"** and **agitated.**
HPI	The patient was diagnosed as suffering from major depressive disorder 1 month ago and had been on an **MAO inhibitor** for 3 weeks. He was switched to **a selective serotonin reuptake inhibitor (SSRI)** last week.
PE	VS: **fever** (39.0°C); **hypertension** (BP 150/100); **tachycardia** (HR 110); **tachypnea** (RR 30). PE: **disoriented; agitated, diaphoretic;** neurologic exam reveals **hyperreflexia, resting** hand **tremor,** and **rigid extremities.**
Labs	ABGs: **metabolic acidosis.**

case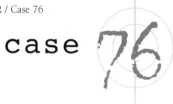

MAO–SSRI Interaction

Differential

Delirium tremens

Neuroleptic malignant syndrome

Sympathomimetic toxicity

Wernicke encephalitis

Discussion

Serotonin syndrome is characterized by an excess of serotonin in the bloodstream. The combination most frequently leading to serotonin syndrome is a **monoamine oxidase (MAO) inhibitor** given with an **SSRI.** Other drugs that can precipitate serotonin syndrome in combination with an MAO inhibitor or an SSRI include **opioids (dextromethorphan, meperidine)** and street drugs such as **cocaine** and **LSD.** In severe cases, serotonin syndrome progresses to **seizures, disseminated intravascular coagulation (DIC), renal failure, coma,** and death. **Tyramine-containing foods,** such as cheeses and beer, in combination with an MAO inhibitor can also cause a hypertensive crisis. Patients should **stop using an MAO inhibitor at least 14 days before starting SSRI** therapy.

Treatment

External cooling; supportive care; IV **benzodiazepines** for agitation and seizures; antihypertensives.

■ TABLE 76-1 EXAMPLES OF INTERACTIONS OF MAO INHIBITORS WITH DRUGS AND FOOD

Type of Interacting Drug	Examples	Outcome	MAO Inhibitor Expected to Interact
Foods containing tyramine (releases norepinephrine)	Cheese, red wine, beer, yeast extracts, aged meats	Hypertension	Nonselective MAO$_A$ selective MAO$_B$ selective
Drugs that release norepinephrine from sympathetic neurons	Amphetamines, ephedrine, phenylpropanolamine, pseudoephedrine	Hypertension	Nonselective MAO$_A$ selective MAO$_B$ selective
Drugs metabolized by monamine oxidase	Phenylephrine (oral)	Hypertension	Nonselective MAO$_A$ selective
	Sumatriptan (Imitrex)	Increased serum levels of sumatriptan	Nonselective MAO$_A$ selective
Drugs that can inhibit serotonin reuptake at synapses	SSRIs, clomipramine (Anafranil), imipramine (Tofranil), meperidine (Demerol), dextromethorphan (Trocal), propoxyphene (Darvon), venlafaxine (Effexor)	Serotonin syndrome, confusion, agitation, hypomania, sweating, myoclonus, fever, coma Can be fatal	Nonselective MAO$_A$ selective MAO$_B$ selective
Serotonin agonists	Sumatriptan	Serotonin syndrome	Nonselective MAO$_A$ selective

MAO$_A$, monoamine oxidase type A; MAOB, monoamine oxidase type B; SSRI, selective reuptake inhibitor.

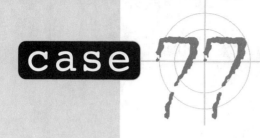

case

ID/CC A 43-year-old art consultant in an advertising agency is brought to the emergency room with **severe headache, palpitations, ringing in her ears,** and **sweating;** she had been **drinking** and dining at a French restaurant.

HPI Over the past several months she had seen several physicians for a variety of complaints before finally being diagnosed with **hypochondriasis** and given medication for it.

PE VS: tachycardia; **hypertension** (BP 180/120); no fever. PE: **pupils dilated;** no papilledema; no signs of long-standing hypertensive retinopathy; no goiter (hyperthyroidism may lead to hypertensive crises).

Labs CBC/Lytes: normal. LFTs normal; no vanillylmandelic acid in urine (seen in pheochromocytoma). UA: normal.

Imaging CXR: normal.

case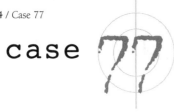

MAO Inhibitor Hypertensive Crisis

Differential

Hypertensive emergency
Pheochromocytoma
Myocardial infarction
Thyroid storm
Amphetamine toxicity

Discussion

Monoamine oxidase (MAO) is an enzyme that degrades catecholamines. When inhibited, catecholamine and serotonin levels increase. MAO inhibitors such as **tranylcypromine** and **phenelzine** are used to treat **anxiety, hypochondriasis,** and **atypical depressions. Tyramine** is a catecholamine food precursor (normally degraded by monoamine oxidase) found in **fermented meats, cheeses, beer, and red wine.** When taken together, tyramine and MAO inhibitors rapidly elevate blood pressure with possible encephalopathy and stroke.

Treatment

Gastric lavage; activated charcoal; treat hypertensive crisis with alpha-blockers to avoid producing hypotension; external cooling to manage hyperthermia. Avoid tyramine-containing foods.

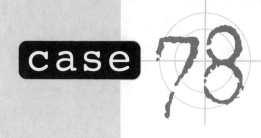

ID/CC   A 27-year-old woman is brought to the emergency room by her mother because of a **high fever** and **muscle rigidity.**

HPI   The patient's mother reports that her daughter is being treated with **antipsychotics** for schizophrenia but is otherwise in good health.

PE   VS: **tachycardia** (HR 165); **hypotension** (BP 100/50); **fever.** PE: **confused** with an altered level of consciousness; pallor; **diaphoresis** (due to autonomic instability); marked rigidity of all muscle groups.

Labs   CBC: **leukocytosis. Increased CK** (indicates muscle damage). ABGs: metabolic **acidosis.**

case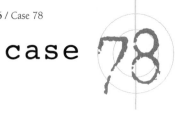

Neuroleptic Malignant Syndrome

Differential

Herpes simplex encephalitis

Rhabdomyolysis

Serotonin syndrome

Lethal catatonia

Dystonic reaction

Cocaine use

Discussion

Neuroleptic malignant syndrome is a life-threatening complication characterized by generalized rigidity and high fever that occur in certain patients with an idiosyncratic reaction to antipsychotics, such as haloperidol and trifluoperazine hydrochloride. The onset of symptoms is usually within a couple of weeks after the drug is started; diminished iron reserves and dehydration are predisposing factors.

Treatment

Treat muscle rigidity with **diazepam** and **initiate rapid cooling** to prevent brain damage (fever may reach dangerous levels). **Dantrolene, dopamine** agonists (bromocriptine) may be effective. Respiratory support.

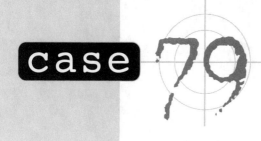

case 79

ID/CC   A 32-year-old man, the lead drummer of a popular rock band, presents to the emergency room with **high fever, running nose,** and **severe diarrhea** as well as abdominal pain.

HPI   He is a chronic user of multiple drugs for 2 years until 2 days ago, when he decided to quit.

PE   VS: **tachycardia** (HR 165); **hypertension** (BP 160/90). PE: patient has **lacrimation and rhinorrhea** and is thin, **anxious,** malnourished, and **sweating** profusely; generalized **piloerection** ("GOOSEBUMPS"); abdomen shows tenderness to deep palpation, but no muscle rigidity or peritoneal signs.

Labs   CBC/Lytes: normal.

case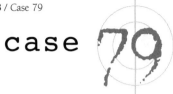

Opiate Withdrawal

Differential | Upper respiratory infection
Gastroenteritis
Influenza
Panic attack
Anxiety disorder

Discussion | Tolerance to opioids is a true cellular adaptive response on many levels, including Ca^{2+} flux, G-protein synthesis, and adenyl cyclase inhibition. Withdrawal effects consist of **rhinorrhea, yawning, piloerection, lacrimation, diarrhea, vomiting, anxiety,** and **hostility.** These effects begin within 6 hours of the last dose and may last 4 to 5 days. Cravings for opiates may last for many years.

Treatment | Treat volume deficit and electrolyte abnormalities resulting from diarrhea; **methadone** for symptomatic relief; **clonidine** to treat sympathetic hyperactivity; **benzodiazepines** for anxiety.

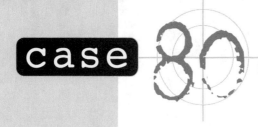

case 80

ID/CC A 52-year-old college professor with a history of **schizophrenia** presents with **tremor and rigidity**.

HPI The patient is **diabetic** and a **smoker** and has been receiving **antipsychotic** therapy for **many years**.

PE **Abnormal facial gestures**, including **lip smacking, jaw muscle spasms,** and jerky movements around mouth; increased blinking frequency and difficulty with speech.

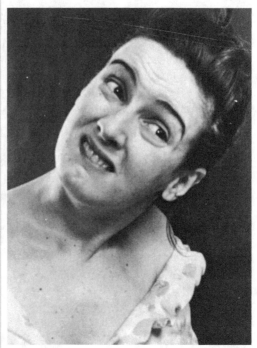

Figure 80-1. Abnormal facial gestures with jaw muscle spasms.

Labs All labs normal.

Imaging XR, skull: calcification of pineal gland.

case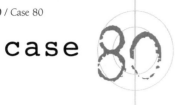

Tardive Dyskinesia

Differential

Huntington disease
Friedreich ataxia
Lesch–Nyhan syndrome
Torticollis
Tourrette syndrome

Discussion

Tardive dyskinesia is a syndrome characterized by late-occurring abnormal **choreoathetoid movements.** It is often associated with antipsychotic drugs (e.g., dopamine blockers) and is estimated to affect about 30% of patients receiving treatment (males and females affected equally). Predisposing factors include older age, smoking, and diabetes. Advanced cases of tardive dyskinesia may be irreversible, so **early recognition of symptoms is critical.**

Treatment

Decreasing dose or switching to atypical neuroleptics is first step. Benzodiazepine treatment can often improve GABAergic activity and therefore alleviate symptoms. Propranolol and calcium channel blockers may be of use.

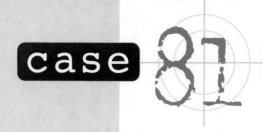

case

ID/CC   A 26-year-old woman is brought to the ER by her boss after **fainting** at work. The day before she had complained of a **dry mouth** along with **constipation and urinary retention**.

HPI   She had a major manic episode of hyperactivity and productivity at work 2 months ago as well as auditory hallucinations, for which she was diagnosed with a **schizoaffective disorder** and has been undergoing treatment with the antipsychotic drug.

PE   VS: **orthostatic hypotension; tachycardia** (HR 108). PE: acute **depression; dryness of mouth;** inability to accommodate normally (with resultant blurred vision); funduscopic exam shows **pigmentary retinopathy** and **dilated pupils;** abdomen slightly distended with diminished peristaltic movements.

Labs   Increased prolactin levels; hyperglycemia. ECG: flattened T-wave; appearance of U-waves; Q-T segment prolongation.

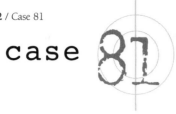

case

Thioridazine Side Effects

Differential | Schizophrenia
Addison disease
Hallucinogen use
Anticholinergic toxicity
Hypothyroidism
Pituitary adenoma

Discussion | Antipsychotic drugs such as thioridazine and chlor-promazine manifest a number of adverse effects, making drug compliance difficult. Muscarinic blockade produces typical anticholinergic effects such as tachycardia, loss of accommodation, urinary retention, and constipation. Alpha blockade produces **orthostatic hypotension.** Other side effects include **extrapyramidal signs** (AKATHISIA, TARDIVE DYSKINESIA, AKINESIA, DYSTONIA, CONVULSIONS). Pigmentary retinopathy is restricted to thioridazine use.

Treatment | Discontinue offending drug.

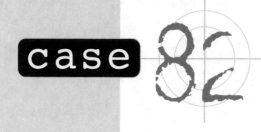

case 82

ID/CC	A 5-year-old boy is rushed to the emergency department after his mother found him playing with her purse, where she carries her **antidepressants;** she noticed that the boy had swallowed a handful of pills.
HPI	The child complained of **dry mouth, blurred vision,** and **hot cheeks** (anticholinergic effect); he also complained of **palpitations** (due to arrhythmias).
PE	VS: tachycardia with irregular rhythm; **fever** (anticholinergic inability to sweat); hypotension. PE: patient **confused;** pupils dilated (MYDRIASIS); **skin warm and red; diminished peristalsis** with no peritoneal signs.
Labs	Lytes: normal. BUN and CPK normal. UA: **myoglobin** present. ECG: occasional premature ventricular contractions (PVCs) and **prolonged QRS** and **QT intervals.**
Imaging	CXR: no pathology found.

case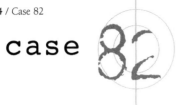

Tricyclic Antidepressant Overdose

Differential

Heart block
Hyperkalemia
Hypocalcemia
Torsades de pointes
Wolff-Parkinson-White syndrome
Digitalis toxicity

Discussion

Tricyclic antidepressants (imipramine, amitriptyline, doxepin) block the reuptake of norepinephrine and serotonin and are used for endogenous depression treatment. TCAs are commonly taken by **suicidal patients** and are a major cause of poisoning and death. Intoxication or overdose may produce **seizures** and **myoclonic jerking** (most common clinical presentation) with **rhabdomyolysis. Death may occur within a few hours.** Other side effects are anticholinergic (**sedation, coma, xerostomia, and diminished bowel sounds**).

Breakout Point

> Tricylic antidepressants (TCAs) are one of the most **commonly overdosed drugs.** Recently, selective serotonin reuptake inhibitors (SSRIs) have decreased the need for this class of potentially lethal agents.

Treatment

Activated charcoal: hemodialysis and hemoperfusion are ineffective owing to large volume of distribution of TCAs: monitor and treat arrhythmias with $NaHCO_3$, lidocaine; treat hypotension with IV fluids or vasopressors if necessary.

case

ID/CC   A 5-year-old boy becomes **cyanotic** and has a **cardiorespiratory arrest** in the ER.

HPI   The child, a known asthmatic, had come to the hospital by ambulance 15 minutes earlier with severe **wheezing, intercostal retractions, nasal flaring, and marked dyspnea.** He was given inhaled anti-inflammatory medications.

PE   Immediate CPR was given, the patient was intubated, and assisted ventilation was administered. The patient came out of the arrest but then returned to his preadmission state of wheezing and respiratory failure.

Labs   CBC: **leukocytosis** (16,000) with neutrophilia. ABGs: mixed respiratory and metabolic acidosis with hypoxemia and hypercapnia. **Peak expiratory flow rate** (PEFR) **markedly reduced** (indicates severe airway obstruction).

Imaging CXR: left lower lobe infiltrate compatible with pneumonia.

case 83

Asthma—Severe Acute

Differential
Airway foreign body
Aspiration
Bronchiolitis
Cystic fibrosis
Bronchopulmonary dysplasia

Discussion
In a severe case of asthma such as this, a preexisting infection is usually the precipitating event. Inhaled steroids have no place in the treatment of an acute attack; as is also the case with sodium cromolyn (cromolyn prevents the release of mast cell mediators, useful for prophylaxis). IV steroids may be given but may take several hours to take full effect (they block leukotriene synthesis by blocking synthesis of phospholipase A2). **Inhaled beta-agonists are the mainstay of acute, emergent therapy** (they activate adenyl cyclase and thereby increase cAMP, which relaxes bronchial smooth muscle). Adverse effects include arrhythmias, tachycardia, and tremors.

Treatment
Metaproterenol by inhalation until bronchospasms stop. Treat infection, acid–base/electrolyte imbalance.

■ TABLE 83-1 RECOMMENDED CHRONIC MEDICATIONS FOR DIFFERENT SEVERITY LEVELS OF ASTHMA

Classification	Short-Term Treatment	Long-Term Treatment	Additional Treatment
Mild–Intermittent	• Short-acting inhaled β_2-agonist • Use of rescue inhaler ≥2 times per week consider long-term treatment	• None needed	• None needed
Mild–Persistent	• Short-acting inhaled β_2-agonist • Use of rescue inhaler daily or increased frequency need additional long-term treatment	• Inhaled low doses of corticosteroids, cromolyn sodium (Intal), or nedocromil (Tilade) • Sustained-release theophylline, zafirlukast	• None needed
Moderate–Persistent	• Short-acting inhaled β_2-agonist • Use of rescue inhaler daily or increased frequency need additional long-term treatment	• Inhaled medium-dose corticosteroids **OR** • Inhaled low-medium dose corticosteroids plus long-acting inhaled β_2-agonist	• Medium-high dose inhaled corticosteroids **AND** • Long-acting inhaled β_2-agonist, sustained-release theophylline, or long-acting β_2-agonist tablets
Severe–Persistent	• Short-acting inhaled β_2-agonist • Use of rescue inhaler daily or increased frequency need additional long-term treatment	• High-dose inhaled corticosteroid **AND** • Long-acting inhaled β_2-agonist, sustained-release theophylline, or long-acting β_2-agonist tablets	• Long-term oral corticosteroids

case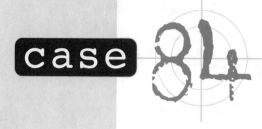

ID/CC A 42-year-old woman presents to her family doctor because of increasing concern over a **facial rash** for the last 2 months that cannot be concealed with cosmetics.

HPI She has also noticed **joint pains** in the knees and sacral region as well as diarrhea. For the past 6 months she has been treated with **an anti-arrhythmic medication** for a supraventricular arrhythmia.

PE Hyperpigmented, brownish **butterfly rash** over the malar region. Left lung is hypoventilated, with dullness to percussion and decreased fremitus (PLEURAL EFFUSION); there is also a pericardial friction rub (due to pericarditis).

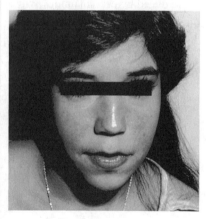

Figure 84-1. Butterfly rash.

Labs **Increased antinuclear antibody (ANA) titer.** Positive antihistone antibodies UA: **proteinuria** (>0.5 mg/dL/day); presence of **cellular casts**. ECG: S-T, T-wave changes (suggestive of pericarditis).

Imaging CXR: small left pleural effusion and enlargement of cardiac silhouette (due to pericardial effusion).

167

case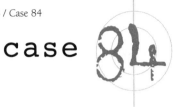

Drug-Induced Lupus

Differential

Systemic lupus erythrematosis

Serum sickness

Preeclampsia

Polyarteritis nodosa

Lyme disease

Discussion

Approximately **one-third of patients** on **long-term procainamide** treatment develop a **lupus-like syndrome.** ANA titer is elevated in nearly all patients receiving this drug, which can also induce **pericarditis, pleuritis,** and pulmonary disease. Other adverse effects include rash, **fever, diarrhea, hepatitis,** and **agranulocytosis.** SLE-like syndrome can also be produced by penicillamine, **hydralazine,** and **isoniazid.**

Treatment

Discontinue procainamide therapy and consider other class IA anti-arrhythmics. Lupus-like symptoms typically resolve.

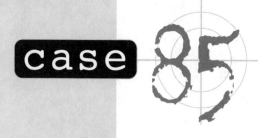

ID/CC   A 30-year-old man is brought to the emergency room in a **stuporous state** with nausea, **protracted vomiting,** and malaise.

HPI   He had been overtreating himself with an analgesic medication with up to 30 pills a day to relieve the pain and discomfort associated with a whiplash neck injury he sustained approximately a week ago.

PE   VS: normal. PE: **icterus; asterixis;** patient **confused** and **dehydrated;** funduscopic exam normal.

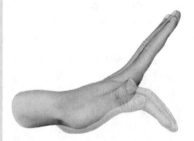

Figure 85-1. Sudden brief nonrhythmic flexion of the hands and fingers indicates asterixis.

TOXICOLOGY

Labs   Markedly **elevated serum transaminases; elevated serum bilirubin; prolonged PT;** mildly elevated serum creatinine and BUN; mild hypoglycemia. ABGs: **metabolic acidosis.**

Imaging   CXR: within normal limits.

Micropathology   Liver biopsy reveals overt coagulative centrilobular necrosis; cells appear shrunken and pyknotic with marked presence of neutrophils.

case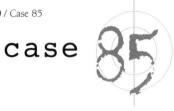

Acetaminophen Overdose

Differential

Gastroenteritis

Hepatitis

Pancreatitis

Amanita mushroom poisoning

Hepatorenal syndrome

Discussion

One of the products of cytochrome P450 metabolism of acetaminophen is hepatotoxic. This reactive metabolite is normally detoxified by glutathione in the liver, but in large doses it may overwhelm the liver's capacity for detoxification. Renal damage may occur because of metabolism by the kidney. Encephalopathy, coma, and death may occur without treatment.

Treatment

N-acetylcysteine as a specific antidote to replete hepatic glutathione levels; supportive management of fulminant hepatic and renal failure; consider liver transplant in severe cases.

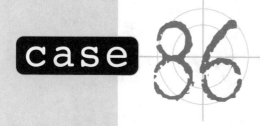

ID/CC A 61-year-old man is admitted to the internal medicine ward for evaluation of **weight loss** and an **increase in abdominal girth.**

HPI He is the father of an African student who is currently studying in the United States. His son brought him here from Central **Africa** for treatment of his disease.

PE Thin, emaciated male; marked **jaundice;** abdomen markedly enlarged due to **ascitic fluid; hepatomegaly;** pitting **edema** in both lower legs.

Labs CBC: anemia (Hb 6.3) (sometimes there may be polycythemia due to ectopic erythropoietin secretion). **Increased α-fetoprotein; hypoglycemia** (due to increased glycogen storage); AST and ALT elevated; alkaline phosphatase elevated.

Imaging US/CT, abdomen: enlargement and enhancement of liver mass with enlargement of regional lymph nodes.

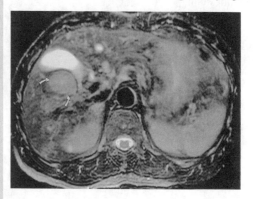

Figure 86-1. Solitary liver mass.

Micropathology Liver biopsy confirms clinical diagnosis, showing fibrotic changes and glycogen accumulation with vacuolation and multinucleated giant cells; pleomorphic hepatocytes seen in a trabecular pattern (may also be adenoid or anaplastic) with malignant change.

171

case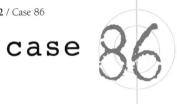

Aflatoxin Carcinogenicity

Differential | Fatty liver
Hepatitis
Hepatic adenoma
Cholangiocarcinoma

Discussion | **Hepatocellular carcinoma** is frequently seen in association with **hepatitis B virus** infections and with cirrhosis. There is a dramatic predisposition to this neoplasia in Africa and in parts of Asia; it is the most common visceral neoplasm in African men. Causative theories include the carcinogenic action of aflatoxins on genetically susceptible individuals and inactivation of the p53 tumor suppressor gene. Aflatoxins are produced by the contamination of peanuts and improperly stored grains (staple food in many African countries) with the fungus *Aspergillus flavus*.

Breakout Point |

> Aflatoxin acts synergistically with hepatitis B virus in the development of hepatocellular carcinoma.

Treatment | Palliative chemotherapy.

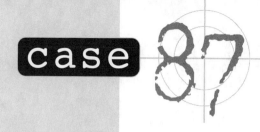

case 87

ID/CC	A 48-year-old factory worker is brought to the ER after a **chemical spill** because of **difficulty breathing** and **irritation of the eyes and throat.**
HPI	He denies allergies, previous surgical operations, diabetes, high blood pressure, infectious diseases, trauma, blood transfusions, and hospitalizations, and he is not on any current medication.
PE	VS: normal. PE: patient conscious, alert, oriented, and in no acute distress; **marked hyperemia** of ocular conjunctiva and upper respiratory passageways; throat mucosa and tongue **edematous** with mucosal **sloughing** on the left side; no laryngospasm; lungs clear to auscultation; abdomen is soft with no masses or peritoneal signs; no focal neurologic signs.
Labs	CBC/Lytes: normal. US: normal.
Imaging	CXR: no evidence of pneumomediastinum.

TOXICOLOGY

case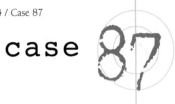

Ammonia Overdose

Differential
Reactive airway disease
Anaphylaxis
Chlorine gas exposure
Hydrogen sulfate exposure
ARDS

Discussion
Ammonia is used as a fertilizer, household chemical, and commercial cleaning agent. Ammonia gas is highly water soluble and produces its **corrosive effects** on contact with tissues such as the eyes and respiratory tract, producing severe laryngitis and tracheitis with possible laryngospasm.

Treatment
Treatment depends on route of exposure to ammonia gas. Observe patient for upper airway obstruction due to inhalation injuries. For eyes and skin, wash exposed regions with water or saline. There are no specific antidotes for this or other caustic burns.

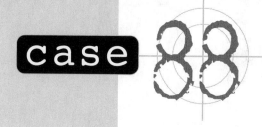

case 88

ID/CC A 10-year-old boy living near a pigment-manufacturing industry presents with a **burning sensation** in a **glove-and-stocking distribution** together with severe **bilateral arm and leg weakness**.

HPI He also presents with **hyperpigmentation** and thickening of the skin over his palms and soles. The child is in the habit of **eating paint**.

PE Hyperkeratosis on palms and soles; peculiar **"raindrop" depigmentation; Aldrich–Mees lines** over nails; neurologic exam reveals decreased sensation, decreased motor strength, absent deep tendon reflexes, and wasting (SYMMETRIC POLYNEUROPATHY) in arms and legs.

Labs Normal.

case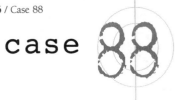

Arsenic Poisoning

Differential

Contact dermatitis

Atopic dermatitis

Guillain–Barré syndrome

Thallium toxicity

Porphyria

Discussion

Arsenic is used in a variety of settings, e.g., as pesticides, herbicides, and rat poison, and in the metallurgic industry. The intoxication may be acute, with violent diarrhea, liver and renal necrosis, and shock potentially leading to death. In chronic exposure, the neurologic symptoms predominate over the gastrointestinal symptoms. The liver and kidney are also affected in chronic exposure.

Breakout Point

> Arsenic inhibits one of the subunits of the pyruvate dehydrogenase complex resulting in impaired production of acetyl-CoA and subsequent oxidative phosphorylation.

Treatment

Chelation with BAL; DMSA, or penicillamine.

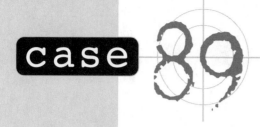

ID/CC A 37-year-old man is brought to the ER by ambulance after collapsing while at work at a **metal-plating** factory.

HPI The factory routinely uses **toxin**-containing compounds in its chemical plating process. A coworker reports that shortly before the patient collapsed, he complained of feeling **nauseated** and having a **headache**.

PE VS: tachycardia (HR 165); hypotension (BP 90/50). PE: patient is experiencing **agonal respiration**, is unresponsive to external stimuli, and exudes a bitter **almond odor**.

TOXICOLOGY

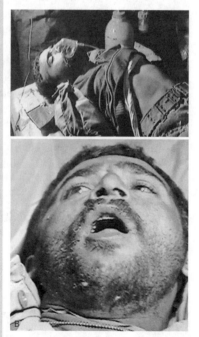

Figure 89-1. Respiratory distress without secretions.

Labs Measured venous oxygen saturation elevated (due to markedly decreased oxygen uptake).

177

case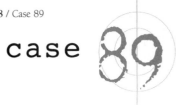

Cyanide Poisoning

Differential

Acute coronary syndrome

Anaphylaxis

Methemoglobinemia

Pulmonary embolism

Strychnine poisoning

Discussion

Cyanide, one of the most powerful poisons known, is a chemical asphyxiant that binds to cytochrome oxidase, blocking the use of oxygen and producing fulminant tissue hypoxia and death in seconds if inhaled or in minutes if ingested. It is used in the photographic, shoe polish, fumigation, and metal-plating industries. Free cyanide is metabolized to thiocyanate, which is less toxic and easily excreted in the urine. Exposure to cyanide gas can be rapidly fatal; however, toxicity due to ingestion of cyanide salts can be slowed with delayed absorption in the GI tract. Administer activated charcoal if accidental oral ingestion is suspected.

Treatment

Treat all cyanide exposure as life-threatening. Give supplemental oxygen. Cyanide antidotes consist of amyl and sodium nitrates, which produce CN-scavenging compounds (especially methemoglobin). Sodium thiosulfate accelerates the conversion of cyanide to thiocyanate.

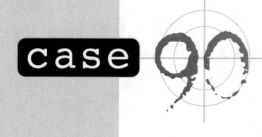

case 90

ID/CC	A 25-year-old man with **HIV/AIDS** complains of severe **shooting pains** in both lower extremities. Pain in the left upper quadrant with radiation to the back.
HPI	The patient is currently taking two **anti-retroviral medications.**
PE	VS: normal. PE: **thin, cachectic** appearance; no evidence of sensory or motor deficits on neurologic exam.
Labs	CBC: leukopenia; elevated MCV (associated with taking reverse transcriptase inhibitors). LFTs mildly elevated. **Serum lipase and amylase** elevated.

case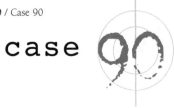

Didanosine Toxicity

Differential

HIV neuropathy

Alcoholism

Gallstone pancreatitis

Pancreatic cancer

Discussion

Didanosine is a nucleoside reverse transcriptase inhibitor used in HAART (highly active antiretroviral therapy) for HIV/AIDS. Its main side effects are **dose-related peripheral neuropathy,** diarrhea, abdominal pain, and **pancreatitis** (1% to 10% risk). Didanosine is also associated with **increased liver enzymes** and **hyperuricemia.** It decreases absorption of numerous antibiotics, including ketoconazole, tetracycline, and fluoroquinolones, and concurrent administration is not recommended.

Treatment

Discontinue ddI and/or d4T and replace with **non-nucleoside reverse transcriptase inhibitor** such as nevirapine. Analgesics, narcotics, tricyclic antidepressants, gabapentin, or alternative therapies such as acupuncture may be effective in treating peripheral neuropathy.

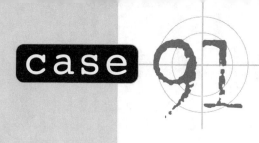

case 97

ID/CC A 2-year-old boy is brought to the emergency room by his mother after a bout of **vomiting**.

HPI The child has been seen by ER staff physicians in the past for **numerous episodes of vomiting and diarrhea.**

PE VS: **tachycardia** (HR 140); mild **hypotension** (BP 100/60). PE: **hyporeflexia; muscle weakness**, and tenderness.

Labs Lytes: serum **potassium low.** BUN, CPK, and creatinine normal. ECG: no arrhythmias or conduction disturbances.

TOXICOLOGY

case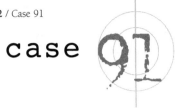

Ipecac Toxicity

Differential

Gastroenteritis

Food allergy

Cystic fibrosis

Inborn error in metabolism

Discussion

Ipecac syrup is an effective drug when induction of vomiting is necessary due to ingestion of drugs and poisons, mainly in children. The safety margin is wide, but deaths have occurred when **fluid extract** of ipecac has been administered (much more concentrated than ipecac syrup). Chronic ipecac poisoning should be suspected in cases in which children are repeatedly brought in with symptoms such as these. Reports of such misuse in cases of "Münchhausen syndrome by proxy" have been recorded. Intoxication may result in cardiomyopathy and fatal arrhythmias (ipecac contains emetine).

Treatment

Treat fluid and electrolyte imbalances. Monitor ECG for changes and possible **arrhythmias** (cause of death).

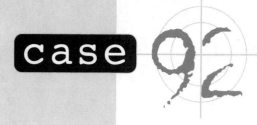
ID/CC   A 5-year-old boy is brought to a medical clinic because of an episode of sudden, **vigorous vomiting** with no previous nausea (PROJECTILE VOMITING) (due to encephalopathy); his mother adds that the child has been **behaving strangely** and has been **irritable**.

HPI   He also complains of **weakness in his hands and feet**. The boy lives in an **old house** that was recently renovated.

PE   Pallor; lethargy; **foot drop** (due to peripheral neuropathy); retinal stippling; lines in gums; **wasting of muscles of hand with motor weakness** (hand grip 50%).

Labs   CBC: **hypochromic, microcytic anemia with basophilic stippling**. Hyperuricemia. UA: **increased urinary coproporphyrin and aminolevulinic acid. Free erythrocyte protoporphyrin levels elevated**; glycosuria; **hypophosphatemia**.

Imaging   XR, long bones: **broad bands** of **increased density** at metaphysis.

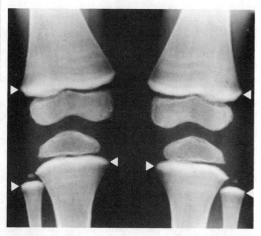

Figure 92-1. Broad bands of increased density at metaphysis.

TOXICOLOGY

case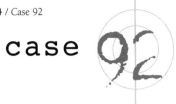

Lead Poisoning

Differential

Acute anemia

Constipation

Mercury toxicity

Intracranial neoplasm

Discussion

Lead poisoning may be caused by gasoline, eating flaking wall paint (as occurs in pica), or using clay utensils with leaded glaze. Poisoning is more common in summer due to sun exposure with increased circulating porphyrins. Lead binds to disulfide groups, causing denaturation of enzymes, and **inhibits ferrochelatase and δ-aminolevulinic acid dehydratase,** thereby interfering with iron utilization in heme synthesis.

Treatment

Separation from source of exposure; chelation therapy with CaEDTA or dimercaprol (IM), or by DMSA (succimer) or penicillamine (oral).

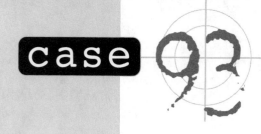
case

ID/CC   A 46-year-old **homeless alcoholic** is brought to the ER by two of his friends in a **confused, incoherent state;** he has been in the ER on many previous occasions.

HPI   He appears unkempt and, as usual, **smells heavily of alcohol.** He complains of nausea, vomiting, and abdominal pain, is very anxious, and constantly repeats that he **cannot see clearly.**

PE   VS: tachycardia; BP normal; **tachypnea** (respiratory compensation to severe acidosis). PE: patient confused as to time, person, and place; speech incoherent; no meningeal or peritoneal signs; no focal neurologic deficit; **marked photophobia** when eye reflex is elicited; papilledema.

Labs   CBC/Lytes: normal. Amylase normal. LFTs: slightly altered (due to chronic alcoholic liver disease). LP: CSF normal. ABGs: **pH 7.2** (ACIDOSIS). **Anion gap increased; serum osmolarity elevated.** ECG: normal.

Imaging   CXR: normal. CT, brain: normal.

Micropathology   Retinal edema with degeneration of ganglion cells; optic nerve atrophy after acute event has subsided.

case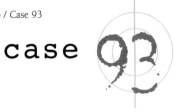

Methanol Poisoning

Differential

Alcohol intoxication

Seizure disorder

Uremia

Hyperammonemia

Subdural hematoma

Discussion

Methyl alcohol (METHANOL) is degraded by dehydrogenase to formaldehyde and formic acid, both of which are toxic compounds that cause a high-anion-gap metabolic acidosis together with ocular lesions that may lead to blindness (due to **retinal and optic nerve atrophy**).

Treatment

Secure airway, breathing, and circulation; for severe acidosis, give sodium bicarbonate; antidote consists of an inhibitor of alcohol dehydrogenase such as **ethanol** or **fomepizole**; provide **folic acid** as a cofactor for formic acid metabolism; consider **hemodialysis** to remove toxin and correct acidosis.

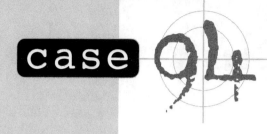

ID/CC A 46-year-old girl scout guide presents to the emergency room of the local rural hospital with excessive **thirst**, weakness, protracted **vomiting**, **acute abdominal pain**, and **severe diarrhea**.

HPI She has been in good health and states that during the camping trip she ate some **wild mushrooms** (about 6 hours ago) that she had hand-picked.

PE VS: **tachycardia** (HR 165); **hypotension** (BP 85/40). PE: lethargy; disorientation; skin is cold and cyanotic; hyperactive bowel sounds on abdominal exam.

Labs **Liver transaminases and bilirubin elevated; PT increased; increased BUN and creatinine.**

Gross Pathology Fulminant hepatitis. **Shrunken liver weighing <500 g. The capsule is baggy** and shrunken away from the liver.

TOXICOLOGY

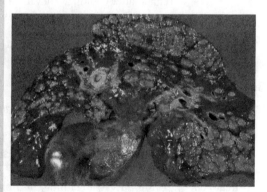

Figure 94-1. Fulminant hepatic failure.

187

case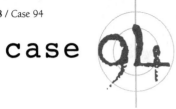

Mushroom Poisoning

Differential

Adrenal crisis

Food allergy

Food poisoning

Isoniazid toxicity

Septic shock

Discussion

There are many species of toxic mushrooms, with clinical pictures varying according to the specific poison involved. Those most commonly involved in the United States are *Amanita phalloides* (delayed intoxication) and *A. muscaria* (rapid toxicity). According to mushroom type, toxins may produce anticholinergic effects (mydriasis, tachycardia, blurred vision) or muscarinic effects (salivation, myosis, bradycardia). These types of mushrooms are often picked and eaten by **amateur foragers.** Toxins are highly stable and remain after cooking. They are absorbed by intestinal cells, and subsequent cell death and sloughing occur within 8 to 12 hours of ingestion. Severe hepatic and renal necrosis is also a common effect of the toxins found in *Amanita phalloides*.

Breakout Point

> The **death cap** (*Amanita phalloides*) mushroom produces α-amanitin, which specifically inhibits eukaryotic RNA-polymerase II, resulting in the termination of mRNA synthesis.

Treatment

Secure airway, breathing, and circulation; if patient presents within 1 hour after ingestion, consider gastric decontamination; thioctic acid may be useful as a free radical scavenger; **high-dose penicillin** blocks hepatic uptake of toxin and increases renal excretion; if hepatic failure ensues, orthotopic **liver transplantation** may be necessary.

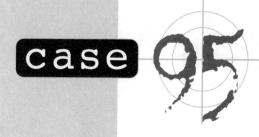

ID/CC A 33-year-old woman with HIV/AIDS presents with a skin **rash**.

HPI Two weeks ago the patient was placed on triple anti-retroviral therapy. She denies fevers, nausea, muscle/joint soreness, headaches, or abdominal pain.

PE VS: normal. PE: **nonpruritic, maculopapular, erythematous rash** diffusely spread across trunk, face, and extremities.

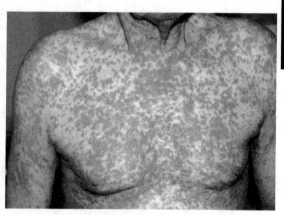

Figure 95-1. Maculopapular rash.

Labs CBC: leukopenia. LFTs mildly elevated.

TOXICOLOGY

189

case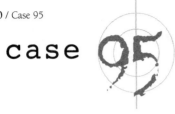

Nevirapine Therapy

Discussion

Nevirapine is a **non-nucleoside reverse transcrip-tase inhibitor (NNRTI)** that directly inhibits HIV reverse transcriptase and is used as part of a 3- or 4-drug regimen to treat HIV. Other NNRTIs include **delavirdine** and **efavirenz**. Side effects of the drug include **rash, fever, nausea, headache,** and **elevations in liver enzymes. Stevens–Johnson syndrome** is a rare but life-threatening complication. Because nevirapine induces **cytochrome P450,** it interacts with many drugs, including cimetidine, fluconazole, ketoconazole, azithromycin, and rifampin; taking such drugs with nevirapine may increase the risk of a rash.

Treatment

Temporarily discontinue or decrease nevirapine dose and, if rash resolves, gradually **dose escalate** nevirapine to reduce risk of recurrence.

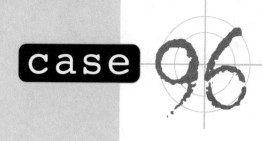

case 96

ID/CC	A 22-year-old white woman who is a professional skier presents to the emergency room complaining of severe **malaise, dizziness,** jaundice, **very low urinary volumes,** and **fatigue.**
HPI	Following a recent skiing accident, in which she sprained her shoulder and knee, she took a total of 20 tablets of an **NSAID** over a 3-day period.
PE	VS: mild hypotension (BP 100/60); no fever. PE: severe dehydration; tenderness to palpation in epigastric area; **pitting ankle and palpebral edema.**
Labs	Lytes: **hyperkalemia.** Markedly **elevated BUN** and **serum creatinine;** urine osmolality increased; fractional excretion of sodium <1%. UA: proteinuria.
Imaging	US, abdomen: normal-sized, normal-appearing kidneys.

TOXICOLOGY

case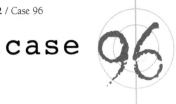

NSAID Toxicity

Differential	Dehydration
	Anemia
	Congestive heart failure
	Acute tubular necrosis
	Mountain sickness
Discussion	Use of NSAIDs, such as diclofenac, can lead to acute renal failure via two mechanisms: (1) unopposed renal vasoconstriction by angiotensin II and norepinephrine; and (2) reduction in cardiac output caused by the associated rise in systemic vascular resistance (an effect that is opposite to the beneficial decrease in cardiac afterload induced by vasodilators). Thus, inhibition of prostaglandin synthesis by an NSAID can lead to **reversible renal ischemia, a decline in glomerular hydrostatic pressure** (the major driving force for glomerular filtration), and **acute renal failure.**
Treatment	Volume replacement, metabolic correction, immediate withdrawal of NSAIDs, avoidance of all nephrotoxic medications.

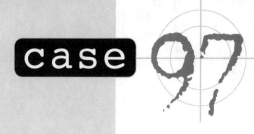

ID/CC   A 28-year-old man comes to his family medicine clinic and complains of **increased bruising** over the past 3 days, as well as **bleeding from the gums** while brushing his teeth.

HPI   The patient is an amateur weight-lifter who recently tried to lift an excessive amount of weight but strained a muscle and has been **taking an NSAID for pain**.

PE   VS: normal. PE: athletic male with significant **ecchymoses** on chest and legs bilaterally; blood pressure cuff leaves petechial lines on arms; blood sample site taken on his arrival for routine blood work has become a large ecchymosis.

Labs   CBC/Lytes/UA: normal. LFTs: normal; **increased PT**.

TOXICOLOGY

case 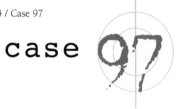 97

NSAID-Induced Qualitative Platelet Disorder

Differential

Hemophilia

Bernard–Soulier syndrome

Glanzmann thrombasthenia

Afibrinogenemia

Discussion

NSAIDs inhibit cyclooxygenase 1 and 2 (COX-1 and COX-2), decreasing prostaglandin production and producing **analgesic, anti-inflammatory, antipyretic,** and **antiplatelet** effects. NSAIDs interfere with platelet function by inhibiting the synthesis of **thromboxane A_2 (TXA_2)**. Aspirin in particular is an irreversible inhibitor, and therefore the production of new platelets (about 8 days) is required before its anticlotting effects can be reversed. Moderate doses of NSAIDs can bring out subclinical platelet defects in otherwise healthy individuals.

Breakout Point

> Genetically inherited qualitative platelet disorders include **Glanzmann thrombasthenia** (a genetic deficiency of platelet glycoprotein IIb/IIIa [GP IIb/IIIa]) and **Bernard–Soulier syndrome** (a genetic deficiency of the glycoprotein Ib).

Treatment

Discontinue indomethacin. Vitamin K may be used in patients with an elevated PT.

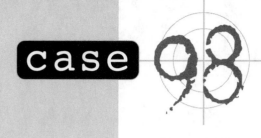

case 98

ID/CC   A 23-year-old woman with **HIV/AIDS** presents to the infectious disease clinic for a regular follow-up.

HPI   She began antiretroviral therapy 1 year ago.

PE   VS: normal. PE: cachectic appearance with peripheral wasting and relative truncal sparing ("**lemon-on-stick**" appearance).

Labs   CBC: normal. Lipid panel reveals **hypercholesterolemia and hypertriglyceridemia; LFTs elevated.**

case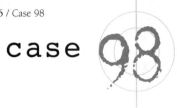

Protease Inhibitor Side Effects

Differential

Corticosteroid use

Kwashiorkor

Discussion

Nelfinavir, ritonavir, indinavir, and **saquinavir** comprise a class of anti-HIV drugs called protease inhibitors. Protease inhibitors are most potent when used as part of a 3- or 4-drug combination in patients who have never previously taken anti-HIV therapies. Side effects include **diarrhea, nausea, rash, lipodystrophy,** and **elevation in liver enzymes. Lipodystrophy** refers to changes in body fat composition that are believed to be related to protease inhibitor use. Other aspects of lipodystrophy include **elevated triglyceride/cholesterol** levels and **hyperglycemia** that can lead to **insulin resistance** and **diabetes.**

Breakout Point

Current treatment recommendations for AIDS include the use of two nucleotide reverse transcriptase inhibitors along with either a non-nucleotide reverse transcriptase inhibitor or a protease inhibitor.

Treatment

Diet, exercise, and **lipid-lowering drugs** to reduce elevated cholesterol/triglyceride levels; monitor for onset of **diabetes;** consider **switching** or **discontinuing protease inhibitors** if necessary. **Human growth hormone** has shown limited benefit in the treatment of lipodystrophy.

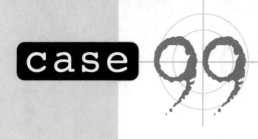

case 99

ID/CC A 5-year-old girl is brought by her parents to the pediatric ER with **severe nausea, hematemesis,** and **abdominal pain.**

HPI She had been playing "candy maker" in her parents' room, and an **open medication bottle** was found on the floor. The child is otherwise healthy.

PE VS: **marked increase in respiratory frequency** (HYPERVENTILATION); **fever;** BP normal. PE: flushed face; lethargy; **disorientation; dehydration; generalized petechiae;** abdominal pain.

Labs CBC: **thrombocytopenia. Elevated PT.** Lytes: normal. ABGs: respiratory alkalosis and metabolic acidosis.

Imaging CXR: within normal limits for age.

case 99

Salicylate Toxicity

Differential
: Diabetic ketoacidosis
Lactic acidosis
Reye syndrome
Iron toxicity

Discussion
: Aspirin toxicity may be pronounced in doses that are only five times the therapeutic amount. Decreased prostaglandin production results in decreased pain, inflammation, and fever. Acute ingestion may affect the integrity of the gastric mucosa and alter blood flow, which are prostaglandin-dependent processes. Diagnosis often depends on patient history, because quantitative levels are often not available. Salicylates stimulate the breathing center, thereby producing hyperventilation and respiratory alkalosis. Salicylates produce a metabolic acidosis as well as ketosis, so at different times during intoxication and depending on the dosage, there will be different, often mixed, acid–base disorders.

Treatment
: If the patient presents early, consider **GI decontamination;** replace fluid losses and correct acid–base disorder; **alkalinize urine** to enhance excretion; if severe, hemodialysis may be necessary; treat gastritis with mucosal protectants, H_2-blockers, or proton pump inhibitors.

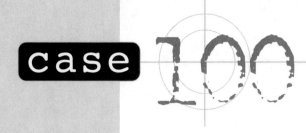

case 100

ID/CC A newborn infant has **underdeveloped limbs** consisting of **short stumps without fingers or toes** (PHOCOMELIA).

HPI Her mother took a drug for erythema nodosum leprosum, a severe complication of leprosy (HANSEN DISEASE) during the first trimester of an unexpected pregnancy.

PE As described.

TOXICOLOGY

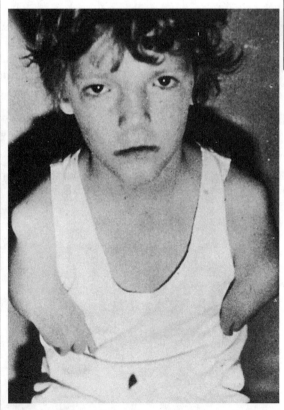

Figure 100-1. Phocomelia (flipper-like appendages).

case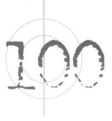

Thalidomide Exposure

Differential

Amniotic band syndrome

Hox gene mutations

Discussion

Thalidomide is a well-known teratogen that was widely used during the first trimester of pregnancy as an agent for insomnia because of its quick sleep-inducing effect. It causes phocomelia, in which a child's limbs resemble the **flippers of a seal,** with failure of development of the long bones of the extremities. Several thousand children were born with this abnormality, making the medical community painfully aware of first-trimester teratogens. Thalidomide induces abortions and multiple other fetal abnormalities. Thalidomide, under highly regulated monitoring, is an effective treatment for complications of leprosy.

Breakout Point

> The use of thalidomide has again surfaced, this time as an anti-cancer agent. It is used primarily in the treatment of multiple myeloma. It is thought to work primarily through inhibiting the production of TNF-α.

questions

1. A 57-year-old man presents to his primary care physician for a regular check-up. A medical student is sent first to gather pertinent history and perform a physical exam. After having reviewed the relevant preventative topics, the student asks the patient if he has any concerns. The patient brings up the fact that he has been having fainting spells at work for the last few months. Upon further questioning, it turns out the patient was started on a new medication for his "heart problems." What medication might be causing the patient's symptoms?

   A. Amiodarone
   B. Propranolol
   C. Captopril
   D. Digitalis
   E. Lidocaine

2. A 60-year-old man is seen in family practice physician's office with a complaint of urinary problems. Patient is being rather vague about his symptoms, and upon delicate questioning it turns out the patient's main concern is really sexual dysfunction. He is very concerned about not being able to achieve an erection, which is a new complaint for him. This started happening about two months ago. The physician looks in the patient's chart and realizes he was started on a new blood pressure medication about two and a half months ago. Which medication could result in the above side effect?

   A. Digitalis
   B. Niacin
   C. Methyldopa
   D. Quinidine
   E. Verapamil

3. A 77-year-old woman presents to her doctor with a request to change the medication she was started on a few weeks ago for treatment of her arrhythmia. She reportedly cannot tolerate the side effects of this new medication, even though her heart palpitations have stopped. Upon review of patient's medications, the physician realizes he started the patient on verapamil. Which combination of side effects could the patient be experiencing?

A. Painful ulcers and fevers
B. Ringing in her ears and headaches
C. Extreme tiredness and fatigability
D. Constipation and facial flushing
E. Chronic dry cough

4. A 23-year-old woman comes to emergency room after she noticed her skin peeling off. She states she has been running high fevers for the last few days, along with difficulty swallowing, so she disregarded her symptoms thinking she had a simple cold. However, she had also noticed she developed a few ulcers in her mouth, and now that her skin started peeling, she decided she should be seen as soon as possible. The patient has been taking some medications for her acne. The constellation of symptoms described in this scenario is referred to as

A. Anabolic steroid abuse
B. Nitrate exposure syndrome
C. Cushing syndrome
D. DES exposure
E. Stevens–Johnson syndrome

5. A 32-year-old woman is diagnosed with rheumatoid arthritis. After a trial of nonsteroidal anti-inflammatory medications, her physician starts the patient on prednisone, because her symptoms are still not well controlled. However, 2 months later, the patient comes back with a request to try a different medication. She feels the side effects of prednisone are not acceptable to her because she works as a flight attendant. Which constellation of side effects is the patient likely to be experiencing?

A. Painful ulcers in mouth and vagina
B. Truncal obesity and moon facies
C. Blurred vision and impaired hearing
D. Facial flushing and itching
E. Objects appearing yellow

6. A 45-year-old man presents to his primary care physician with concerns about his weight. He is 5 feet and 10 inches, and his weight is 290 pounds. The patient has tried losing weight through diet and exercise, but was unsuccessful because he could not follow the strict regimens. He is now interested in getting some information about gastric bypass surgery, but he is afraid of the risks of a surgical procedure. His physician decides to present him with an option of anti-obesity drugs. Which of the following medications might be used to help patients lose weight?

A. Alendronate
B. Megestrol
C. Cimetidine
D. Orlistat
E. Ephedrine

7. A 75-year-old woman who is hospitalized for urosepsis develops profuse diarrhea accompanied by extreme dehydration and decreased mental status. The patient's stool sample is sent for analysis and while the results are still pending, her status deteriorates. She undergoes emergent colonoscopy and the findings are consistent with pseudomembranous colitis. After review of her medications, her medical team finds the responsible agent. Which of the following classes of medications most likely resulted in such dangerous side effect?

A. Anti-arrhythmic
B. Laxative
C. Antibiotic
D. Nonsteroidal anti-inflammatory
E. Weight loss supplement

8. A 47-year-old woman presents to her doctor after having found a lump in her breast during a routine monthly self-exam. The physician confirms the finding and sends the patient for a biopsy. The results come back positive for invasive ductal carcinoma. The patient undergoes lumpectomy, and is then started on chemotherapy. After three cycles, she presents to her oncologist with complaints of shortness of breath at night and frequent fainting spells. After undergoing an echocardiogram, the patient is told she has a mild form of cardiomyopathy. Which of the following chemotherapeutic agents is likely to be the cause of such cardiotoxicity?

A. Doxorubicin
B. Cyclophosphamide
C. Cisplatin
D. Bleomycin
E. Aniline

9. A 28-year-old woman with systemic lupus erythematosis is started on cyclosporine as part of her steroid-sparing regimen. Three months later, her symptoms seem to be well controlled, but she develops some side effects that make her rheumatologist consider alternate regimens. Which of the following side effects did the patient most likely develop?

A. Black tarry stools
B. Ulcerations of the oral mucosa
C. Fevers and muscle aches
D. Elevated blood pressure
E. Increased urinary frequency

10. A 25-year-old college student presents to an urgent care clinic after experiencing several episode of seeing "halos" around lights. Upon gathering thorough history, the nurse practitioner learns the patient has also been experiencing blurry vision and itching while taking a shower. Additionally, it turns out the patient had recently returned from a safari trip to Kenya, for which she was started on a prophylactic medication. Which agent might that be?

A. Amphotericin B
B. Chloramphenicol
C. Chloroquine
D. Fluoroquinolone
E. Gentamicin

11. A 19-year-old man presents to emergency room for an evaluation of rash he developed over the course of several hours. He had gone hiking earlier that day while wearing shorts and sandals without socks. At one point he admits he may have been bitten by a tick; however he did not find one on his skin, so he forgot the incident. The patient's titers are drawn to evaluate him for Lyme disease, and in the meantime he is given a prescription for tetracycline. Which set of side effects is possible with this antibiotic?

A. Red colored urine and orange staining on clothes
B. Fatigue and scleral icterus
C. Hearing loss and vertigo
D. Bleeding from gums
E. Rash on sun-exposed area of body

12. A 26-year-old medical student develops a generalized seizure while studying at home for one of his finals. He has been staying up every night for a week. This is his first seizure, so the neurologist starts him on a new medication. When the patient comes for a follow-up 3 months later, he complains of frequent colds and bleeding from his gums. He also states he has bouts of double vision, as well as occasional feeling of dry mouth. Which of the following medications may this patient have been started on?

A. Phenytoin
B. Carbamazepine
C. Amantadine
D. Levodopa
E. Ketamine

13. A 35-year-old man is brought to the emergency room by his wife after she found him clutching his chest. The patient describes heavy retrosternal pain that radiates to his left arm. His cardiac enzymes are elevated and the ECG shows ST-segment elevation in the inferior leads. Patient is diagnosed with myocardial infarction and admitted to cardiac intensive care unit. He undergoes cardiac catheterization, which reveals normal coronary anatomy. His blood toxicology screen comes back positive for one of the substances of abuse. Which agent might have been at fault in this scenario?

A. Cannabis
B. Heroin
C. LSD
D. PCP
E. Cocaine

14. A 19-year-old man is arrested after a high-speed chase and an attempted robbery of a local gas station. His roommate reports that his friend has been acting funny lately. He has been sleeping less and talking very fast. He has also been spending huge amounts of money. The young man is evaluated by the police psychologist, who determines that he likely has bipolar disorder. The man is referred to a psychiatrist, who admits him to a recovery hospital and starts him on a mood-stabilizing medication. Several days later, the patient develops increased uncontrollable thirst and frequent urination. He also complains of severe acne. Which medication did this patient start taking?

A. Lithium
B. Clozapine
C. Carbamazepine
D. Methylphenidate
E. Phenelzine

15. A concerned mother brings her 4-year-old son to a pediatrician. She states that the boy has been having attacks of sudden vomiting. He has also been complaining of frequent episodes of abdominal pain. Upon further questioning, it is revealed the patient has been very irritable lately, and has complained of weakness in his hands and feet. The family of the boy lives in an old apartment in a not very desired part of town. Pediatrician suspects the boy is probably suffering from poisoning. Which substance is the most likely offending agent?

A. Iron
B. Lead
C. Arsenic
D. Cyanide
E. Ammonia

16. A 55-year-old man presents to cardiologist for a routine follow-up. He suffers from a supraventricular arrhythmia, for which he was recently started on a new medication. On exam, the patient is found to have a brownish malar rash, joint tenderness, and a pericardial friction rub. Which of the following medication is the most likely cause of such symptoms?

A. Bleomycin
B. Captopril
C. Methyldopa
D. Procainamide
E. Furosemide

17. A 32-year-old man presents to an urgent care clinic with severe cold that has lasted for over a week. Patient complains of a runny nose and a sore throat that has now progressed to persistent cough. On exam, the patient is found to have several enlarged lymph nodes and oral thrush. His blood samples are sent for several tests and a week later, the patient receives a call urging him to follow up in the clinic. The patient is told he is HIV positive. He is referred to a support group and an infectious disease specialist. After running the test to determine the patient's CD4 count and viral load, the infectious disease specialist starts the patient on an antiretroviral regimen. However, a month later the patient comes back complaining of shooting pains in his legs. Which medication might be causing this side effect?

A. Nevirapine
B. Indinavir
C. Saquinavir
D. Didanosine
E. Amantadine

18. A 5-year-old girl is brought to the emergency room after her mother found her lethargic and hyperventilating. Upon questioning of the child, the emergency physician finds out the patient is also suffering from severe nausea and abdominal pain. An arterial blood gas is sent urgently and comes back revealing respiratory alkalosis and metabolic acidosis. Which of the following might this child have ingested?

NSAIDs
Salicylates
Mushrooms
Lead
Methanol

7-year-old boy is brought to the emergency room after his brother found him gasping for air. The boy suffers from asthma, but his parents have not been following the plan outlined by their pediatrician. The boy was supposed to take his steroid inhaler every day, and use his bronchodilator inhaler only when needed. As it turns out, the patient has not been taking his inhaled steroids at all because he never remembered to do so, and his parents failed to remind him. Which medication should be administered urgently to stop this patient's acute bronchospasm?

A. Prednisone
B. Chromolyn
C. Metaproterenol
D. Theophylline
E. Penicillin

20. A 44-year-old woman who suffers from major depressive disorder presents to an urgent care clinic with complaints of fever, dry mouth, and blurred vision. She has been taking her medications as usual up until a few days ago, when she decided her symptoms were not well controlled, so she increased her medication dose several times. After a long talk, the patient finally agrees to check into a psychiatric recovery hospital to gain better control of her symptoms. Which of the following phenomena is described in this vignette?

A. MAOI–SSRI interaction
B. Tardive dyskenisia
C. Malignant hyperthermia
D. Tricyclic overdose
E. Neuroleptic malignant syndrome

answers

1-B

    A. Amiodarone [INCORRECT] may cause unexplained fatigue and anxiety.

    B. Propranolol [CORRECT], as demonstrated in this vignette, can cause fainting spells, dizziness, and dyspnea.

    C. Captopril [INCORRECT], an ACE inhibitor, can cause chronic dry cough.

    D. Digitalis [INCORRECT] can cause headaches, lethargy, and can make objects appear yellow.

    E. Lidocaine [INCORRECT] injected into the bloodstream can cause seizures.

2-C

    A. Digitalis [INCORRECT] can cause nausea, vomiting, and visual disturbances.

    B. Niacin [INCORRECT] can cause facial flushing.

    C. Methyldopa [CORRECT] can result in sexual side effects, as is described in this scenario.

    D. Quinidine [INCORRECT] can cause tinnitus and GI distress.

    E. Verapamil [INCORRECT] can cause constipation.

3-D

    A. Painful ulcers and fevers [INCORECT] are characteristic of Stevens–Johnson syndrome.

    B. Ringing in one's ears and headaches [INCORRECT] may be caused by quinidine.

    C. Methyldopa can cause extreme tiredness and fatigability [INCORRECT].

    D. Verapamil, the source of the problems for this patient, can cause facial flushing and constipation [CORRECT].

    E. Chronic dry cough [INCORRECT] can be caused by ACE inhibitors, such as captorpil.

4-E

    A. Anabolic steroid abuse [INCORRECT] can result in impotence and labile behavior.

    B. Nitrate exposure [INCORRECT] is characterized by chronic headaches and dizziness.

C. Cushing syndrome [INCORRECT] is characterized by truncal obesity, moon facies, purple stria, and other undesirable side effects.

D. DES exposure in utero [INCORRECT] can result in clear cell adenocarcinoma of the vagina.

E. Stevens–Johnson syndrome [CORRECT], described in this vignette, is a life-threatening condition characterized by high fevers and skin desquamation.

5-B

A. Painful ulcers in mouth and vagina [INCORRECT] can be a sign of Stevens–Johnson syndrome.

B. Truncal obesity and moon facies [CORRECT] are side effects of exogenous corticosteroid use, as is described in this scenario.

C. Blurred vision and impaired hearing [INCORRECT] can be caused by quinidine.

D. Facial flushing and itching [INCORRECT] can be caused by verapamil.

E. Digitalis can cause objects to appear yellow [INCORRECT] as one of its side effects.

6-D

A. Alendronate [INCORRECT] is a bisphosphonate used for prevention of osteoporosis.

B. Megestrol [INCORRECT] can be used as an appetite stimulant for patient with cancer and AIDS.

C. Cimetidine [INCORRECT] is an H2-blocker used for peptic ulcer disease and GERD.

D. Orlistat [CORRECT] can be used as a weight loss aide if patients are unsuccessful in losing weight through diet and exercise.

E. Ephedrine [INCORRECT] can cause worsening of anginal symptoms.

7-C

A. Anti-arrhythmic medications [INCORRECT] are not known to result in pseudomembranous colitis. Many can cause additional arrhythmias, so close monitoring is warranted.

B. Laxatives [INCORRECT] can cause diarrhea, but they will not cause pseudomembranous colitis.

C. Antibiotics [CORRECT] are well known for causing pseudomembranous colitis due to alterations in gut flora. Most common antibiotics associated with this dangerous condition are cephalosporins and clindamycin.

    D. Non-steroidal anti-inflammatory agents [INCORRECT] can cause peptic ulcer disease.

    E. Weight-loss supplements such as orlsitat [INCORRECT] can have diarrhea as one of their side effects, but they would not cause pseudomembranous colitis.

8-A

    A. Doxorubicin, [CORRECT] a part of some chemotherapeutic regimens used for breast cancer, is known for causing cardiotoxicity, particularly cardiomyopathy, as is demonstrated in this vignette.

    B. Cyclophosphamide [INCORRECT] can result in hemorrhagic cystitis.

    C. Cisplatin [INCORRECT] can cause decreased auditory acuity.

    D. Bleomycin [INCORRECT] can result in pulmonary fibrosis.

    E. Aniline dye exposure [INCORRECT] can result in bladder cancer.

9-D

    A. Black tarry stools [INCORRECT], a manifestation of GI bleeding, can be caused by warfarin.

    B. Ulcerations of the oral mucosa [INCORRECT] can result from use of methotrexate.

    C. Fevers and muscle aches [INCORRECT] are characteristic of interferon use.

    D. Cyclosporine, a commonly used immunosuppressant, can result in hypertension [CORRECT], as described in this scenario.

    E. Increased urinary frequency and dysuria [INCORRECT] can be early signs of hemorrhagic cystitis.

10-C

    A. Amphotericin B [INCORRECT] can cause high fever, marked lightheadedness, headache, and myalgias.

    B. Chloramphenicol [INCORRECT] can cause recurrent infections (neutropenia), excessive bleeding (thrombocytopenia) and malaise, weakness, and apathy (anemia).

    C. Chloroquine [CORRECT], an antimalarial medication, can result in visual disturbances, as described in this vignette ("halos" around lights).

    D. Elevated blood pressure can result form many medications, particularly cyclosporine [INCORRECT].

    E. Increased urinary frequency is commonly seen with cyclophosphamide use [INCORRECT].

11-E

    A. Red-colored urine and orange staining [INCORRECT] on clothes is seen with rifampin use.

    B. Fatigue and scleral icterus [INCORRECT], signs of hepatitis, can be seen with INH use.

    C. Gentamicin is an ototoxic agent, and can result in hearing loss and vertigo [INCORRECT].

    D. Bleeding from gums [INCORRECT] can be seen with chloramphenicol use as a result of thrombocytopenia.

    E. Tetracycline, the offending agent in this question, can result in development of rash on sun-exposed areas of body [CORRECT], especially in fair-skinned individuals.

12-B

    A. Phenytoin [INCORRECT] can result in tremors, dizziness, inability to walk properly, and double vision.

    B. Carbamazepine [CORRECT] can cause neutropenia (frequent colds) and thrombocytopenia (bleeding from gums), as well as double vision, ataxic gait, and sleepiness.

    C. Amantadine [INCORRECT] can cause dizziness and vertigo.

    D. Levodopa [INCORRECT] can cause tremors and dyskenisia.

    E. Ketamine [INCORRECT] can result in vivid hallucinations.

13-E

    A. Cannabis (marijuana) [INCORRECT] can cause mild somnolence, stupor, and motor dysfunction.

    B. Heroin [INCORRECT] can result in tonic-clonic seizures; respiratory depression; stupor; pinpoint pupils; and marked hyporeflexia.

    C. LSD [INCORRECT] can result in vivid hallucinations.

    D. PCP [INCORRECT] can cause volatile behaviors and hallucinations.

    E. Cocaine overdose [CORRECT] results in coronary vasospasm, and in severe cases, as described in this vignette, can cause myocardial infarction.

14-A

    A. Lithium [CORRECT], a commonly used mood stabilizer used for treatment on bipolar disorder, can cause polydipsia, polyuria, as well as severe acne.

    B. Clozapine [INCORRECT] can occasionally cause agranulocytosis.

    C. Carbamazepine [INCORRECT] can cause neutropenia and thrombocytopenia.

D. Methylphenidate [INCORRECT] can cause restlessness, euphoria, anxiety, tachycardia, paranoia, and agitation.

E. Phenelzine [INCORRECT] is an MAOI, and its use in conjunction with tyramine-containing foods can result in hypertensive crisis.

15-B

A. Iron overdose [INCORRECT] can cause diarrhea and bluish-green emesis.

B. Lead poisoning [CORRECT] can result in abdominal pain and peripheral neuropathy, as is the case with the child described in this vignette.

C. Arsenic poisoning [INCORRECT] can result in symmetric polyneuropathy in arms and legs.

E. Cyanide poisoning [INCORRECT] can be life-threatening and is usually preceded by nausea and headaches.

F. Ammonia overdose [INCORRECT] can present with difficulty breathing and irritation of the eyes and throat.

16-D

A. Bleomycin [INCORRECT] use can result in pulmonary fibrosis.

B. Captorpil's [INCORRECT] side effects can include dry cough.

C. Methyldopa [INCORRECT] can cause sexual dysfunction.

D. Procainamide [CORRECT] can cause drug-induced lupus, as presented in this case, with malar rash and arthralgia.

E. Furosemide [INCORRECT], a loop diuretic, can cause hypokalemic metabolic alkalosis.

17-D

A. Nevirapine [INCORRECT] can cause nonpruritic, macu-lopapular, erythematous rash.

B. Indinavir [INCORRECT] can cause cachectic appearance with peripheral wasting and relative truncal sparing.

C. Saquinavir [INCORRECT], another example of protease inhibitor can cause side effects mentioned in choice B.

D. Didanosine [CORRECT] can result in dose-related peripheral neuropathy, diarrhea, abdominal pain, and pancreatitis; peripheral neuropathy can mimic sciatica-type pain in presentation.

E. Amantadine [INCORRECT] can result in cerebellar problems such as ataxic gait, slurred speech, and dizziness.

18-B

    A. NSAID overdose [INCORRECT] can lead to reversible renal ischemia and acute renal failure.

    B. Salicylate intoxication [CORRECT] can present as marked increase in respiratory frequency; fever; lethargy; disorientation; dehydration; and generalized petechiae. ABG would show respiratory alkalosis and metabolic acidosis.

    C. Mushroom poisoning [INCORRECT] can present either with anticholinergic or muscarinic effects.

    D. Lead poisoning [INCORRECT] can cause peripheral neuropathy.

    E. Methanol poisoning [INCORRECT] can lead to retinal and optic nerve atrophy.

19-C

    A. Prednisone [INCORRECT], a steroid medication, is not used for acute treatment of asthmatic attack.

    B. Chromolyn [INCORRECT] prevents the release of mast cell mediators and is useful for prophylaxis of asthma.

    C. Metaproterenol [CORRECT] is a beta-agonist and is the mainstay of acute, emergent therapy. It activates adenyl cyclase and thereby increases cAMP, which relaxes bronchial smooth muscle.

    D. Theophylline [INCORRECT] is a methylxanthine that works for nocturnal asthma treatment via slow release preparation by inhibition of adenosine receptor.

    E. Penicillin [INCORRECT] is an antibiotic and has no place in treatment of acute bronchospasm.

20-D

    A. MAOI–SSRI interaction [INCORRECT], known as serotonin syndrome, can present as seizures, disseminated intravascular coagulation (DIC), renal failure, coma, and in severe cases, death.

    B. Tardive dyskenisia [INCORRECT] is characterized by late-occurring abnormal choreoathetoid movements.

    C. Malignant hyperthermia [INCORRECT] can present with tachycardia, hypertension, acidosis, hyperkalemia, and muscle rigidity, and it appears to be related to excess myoplasmic calcium.

    D. Tricyclic antidepressant overdose [CORRECT] can present with fever, dry mouth, and blurred vision; however, it can quickly progress to seizures and myoclonic jerking with rhabdomyolysis. In most severe cases, such overdose may be fatal.

    E. Neuroleptic malignant syndrome [INCORRECT] is a life-threatening complication, characterized by generalized rigidity and high fever, that occurs in certain patients with an idiosyncratic reaction to antipsychotics.

credits

Becker KL, Bilezikian JP, Brenner WJ, et al. *Prinicples and Practice of Endocrinology and Metabolism*, 3rd ed. Philadelphia: Lippincott Williams & Wilkins; 2001. Figs. 75-6 B&C (Case 13), 115-2 (Case 22), 80-10 (Case 53).

Billings RJ, Berkowitz RJ, Watson G. Moderate tetracycline staining. *Teeth Pediatrics* 2004;113:1120–1127. Fig. 2 (Case 51).

Eisenberg RL. *Clinical Imaging: An Atlas of Differential Diagnosis*, 4th ed. Philadelphia: Lippincott Williams & Wilkins; 2002. Figs. B 2-1 (Case 16), C 9-1 B (44-1), B20-1 (Case 92).

Fleisher GR, Ludwig S, Baskin MN. *Atlas of Pediatric Emergency Medicine*. Phildelphia: Lippincott Williams & Wilkins; 2004. Fig. 15.15 (Case 70).

Gillenwater JY, Grayhack JT, et al. *Adult and Pediatric Urology*, 4th ed. Philadelphia: Lippincott Williams & Wilkins; 2001. Fig. 6.9A (Case 29).

Golan DE, Tashijian AH, et al. *Principles of Pharmacology: The Pathophysiologic Basis of Drug Therapy.* Philadelphia: Lippincott Williams & Wilkins, 2005. Table 30-2. (Case 44)

Goodheart HP. *Goodheart's Photoguide of Common Skin Disorders*, 2nd ed. Philadelphia: Lippincott Williams & Wilkins; 2003. Fig. 2.63 (Case 84).

Grammer LC, Greenberger PA. *Patterson's Allergic Diseases*, 6th ed. Philadelphia: Lippincott Williams & Wilkins; 2002. Fig. 16.5 (Case 11).

Greenberg MJ, Hendrickson RG. *Greenberg's Text-Atlas of Emergency Medicine*. Philadelphia: Lippincott, Williams & Wilkins; 2004. Figs. 7-39 (Case 2), 33-3 (Case 21), 24-11 (Case 35), 7-6A (Case 66), 30-17 (Case 89), 24-51A (Case 95).

Greer JP, Foerster J, Lukens J, et al. *Wintrobe's Clinical Hematology*, 11th ed. Philadelphia: Lippincott Williams & Wilkins; 1998. Figs. 27.18.C (Case 6), 49.1 (Case 8), 44.1 (Case 42).

Humes HD, DuPont HL, Gardner LB, et al. *Kelley's Textbook of Internal Medicine*, 4th ed. Philadelphia: Lippincott Williams & Wilkins; 2000. Figs. 76.9 (Case 4), 197.1 (Case 48).

Jacob LS. *NMS Pharmacology.* 4th ed. Media, PA: Williams & Wilkins, 1996: Table 10-3. (Case 12)

Kelson DP, Daly JM, et al. *Gastrointestinal Oncology: Principles and Practice.* Philadelphia: Lippincott Williams & Wilkins; 2002. Fig. 10.15A (Case 86).

Porth CM. *Pathophysiology Concepts in Altered Health States,* 6th ed. Philadelphia: Lippincott Williams & Wilkins; 2002. Fig. 34.1 (Case 23).

Rowland LP. *Merritt's Neurology,* 11th ed. Philadelphia: Lippincott Williams & Wilkins; 2005. Fig. 113.3 (Case 80).

Rubin E, Farber JL. *Pathology,* 3rd ed. Philadelphia: Lippincott Williams & Wilkins; 1999. Fig. 16.76 (Case 55).

Rubin E, Gorstein F, Schwarting R, et al. *Rubin's Pathology: A Clinicopathologic Approach.* 4th ed. Baltimore: Lippincott Williams & Wilkins; 2004. Figs. 8-17 (Case 15), 8-27 (Case 20), 8-12 (Case 74), 14-27A (Case 94), 6-6 (Case 100).

Sadler T. *Langman's Medical Embryology,* 9th ed. Image Bank. Baltimore: Lippincott Williams & Wilkins; 2003. Fig. 6.8B (Case 60).

Sadock BJ, Sadock VA. *Kaplan & Sadock's Comprehensive Textbook of Psychiatry.* 8th ed. Philadelphia: Lippincott Williams & Wilkins; 2005: Table 31.19-3. (Case 76)

Saenz RE, Sears BW, Dabisch PA. *Hardcore Pharmacology.* Baltimore: Lippincott Williams & Wilkins: T4-9. (Case 7).

Saenz RE, Sears BW, Dabisch PA. *Hardcore Pharmacology.* Philadelphia: Lippincott Williams & Wilkins; 2005. Figs. 4-11 (Case 3), 4-9 (Case 7), Table 9-1 (Case 31).

Schiff ER, Sorrell MF, Maddrey WC. *Schiff's Diseases of the Liver,* 9th ed. Philadelphia: Lippincott Williams & Wilkins; 2003. Fig. 56.9 (Case 28).

Scott JR, Gibbs RS, et al. *Danforth's Obstetrics and Gynecology,* 9th ed. Philadelphia: Lippincott Williams & Wilkins; 2003. Fig. 16.5 (Case 11).

Smith C, Marks A, Lieberman M. *Mark's Basic Medical Biochemistry: A Clinical Approach,* 2nd ed. Philadelphia: Lippincott Williams & Wilkins; 2004. Fig. 40.5 (Case 36).

Topol EJ, Califf RM, Isner J, et al. *Textbook of Cardiovascular Medicine*, 2nd ed. Philadelphia: Lippincott Williams & Wilkins; 2002. Figs. 37.3 (Cases 1 & 2), 90.1 (Case 33), 59.6 (Case 72).

Weber J, Kelley J. *Health Assessment in Nursing*, 2nd ed. Philadelphia: Lippincott Williams & Wilkins; 2003. Fig. 15.12 (Case 47).

Yamada T, Alpers DH, et al. *Textbook of Gastroenterology*, 4th ed. Philadelphia: Lippincott Williams & Wilkins; 2003. Figs. 85-4 (Case 26), 88-2 (Case 27).

case list

CARDIOLOGY
1. Amiodarone Side Effects
2. Beta-Blocker Overdose
3. Captopril Side Effects
4. Digitalis Intoxication
5. Lidocaine Toxicity
6. Methyldopa Side Effects
7. Niacin Side Effects
8. Nitrate Exposure
9. Quinidine Side Effects
10. Verapamil Side Effects

DERMATOLOGY
11. Stevens–Johnson Syndrome

ENDOCRINOLOGY
12. Anabolic Steroid Abuse
13. Cushing's Syndrome—Iatrogenic
14. Diethylstilbestrol (DES) Exposure
15. Oral Contraceptive Side Effects
16. Osteoporosis Prophylaxis—Hormonal
17. Osteoporosis Prophylaxis—Nonhormonal
18. Osteoporotic Fracture—Bisphosphonates

GASTROENTEROLOGY
19. Alternative Pharmacotherapy
20. Anorectic/Anti-obesity Agents
21. Appetite Stimulants—Megestrol/THC
22. Cimetidine Side Effects
23. Hemorrhagic Gastritis—Drug-induced
24. Hepatitis—Halothane
25. Hepatitis—INH
26. Laxative Abuse
27. Pseudomembranous Colitis
28. Reye's Syndrome

HEMATOLOGY/ONCOLOGY
29. Aniline Dye Carcinogenicity
30. Bleomycin Toxicity
31. Cisplatin Side Effects
32. Cyclophosphamide Side Effects
33. Doxorubicin Cardiotoxicity
34. Heparin Overdose
35. Iron Overdose
36. Methotrexate Toxicity
37. Warfarin Interactions
38. Warfarin Toxicity

IMMUNOLOGY
39. Cyclosporine Side Effects
40. Interferon Use

INFECTIOUS DISEASE
41. Amphotericin B Toxicity
42. Chloramphenicol Side Effects
43. Chloroquine Toxicity
44. Drug Resistance
45. Fluoroquinolone Side Effects
46. Gentamicin Side Effects
47. Ketoconazole Side Effects
48. Penicillin Allergic Reaction
49. Rifampin Side Effects
50. Tamiflu Therapy
51. Tetracycline Side Effects
52. Zidovudine Toxicity

NEPHROLOGY/UROLOGY

53. Loop Diuretic Side Effects
54. Thiazide Side Effects
55. Tubulointerstitial Disease—
    Drug-induced
56. Viagra (Sildenafil) Therapy

NEUROLOGY

57. Amantadine Toxicity
58. Anticonvulsant Osteomalacia
59. Carbamazepine Side Effects
60. Fetal Alcohol Syndrome
61. Ketamine Side Effects
62. Levodopa Side Effects
63. Malignant Hyperthermia
64. Parkinson Disease—MPTP-
    induced
65. Phenytoin Overdose

ORTHOPEDICS

66. COX-II Inhibitors

PSYCHOPHARMACOLOGY

67. Amphetamine Abuse
68. Amphetamine Withdrawal
69. Barbiturate Intoxication
70. Cannabis Intoxication
71. Clozapine Toxicity
72. Cocaine Abuse
73. Cocaine Withdrawal
74. Heroin Overdose
75. Lithium Side Effects
76. MAO-SSRI Interaction

77. MAO Inhibitor Hypertensive
    Crisis
78. Neuroleptic Malignant Syndrome
79. Opiate Withdrawal
80. Tardive Dyskinesia
81. Thioridazine Side Effects
82. Tricyclic Antidepressant
    Overdose

PULMONARY

83. Asthma—Severe Acute

RHEUMATOLOGY

84. Drug-induced Lupus

TOXICOLOGY

85. Acetaminophen Overdose
86. Aflatoxin Carcinogenicity
87. Ammonia Overdose
88. Arsenic Poisoning
89. Cyanide Poisoning
90. Didanosine Toxicity
91. Ipecac Toxicity
92. Lead Poisoning
93. Methanol Poisoning
94. Mushroom Poisoning
95. Nevirapine Therapy
96. NSAID Toxicity
97. NSAID-induced Qualitative
    Platelet Disorder
98. Protease Inhibitor Side Effects
99. Salicylate Toxicity
100. Thalidomide Exposure

index